Eternal Yoga
Awakening within Buddhic Consciousness

Preface

This book holds keys for advancing upon the spiritual path into a conscious continuum beyond the temporary limits of birth and death, therefore assuring victory in our eternal nature. The true understanding of these keys becomes alive through our radiant communion with those who have victoriously applied them, the Ascended Masters.

In our modern culture and time, most have no idea of what the spiritual path really is, confusing it with morality, ambitions, emotions, sensations, scriptures, and religions. Those who see through this confusion, in their subsequent rebellion, will often cast aside the sacred, proclaiming their divinity in independence, and thus further lose their self in separation.

We need ways to gain direct experience of the enlightened view, so that, within our heart, we exist beyond separation and through our eyes, we see underneath separation. In this way, a healing occurs whereby we also see the perfection of apparent separation itself. This non-dual view, we call the natural state.

The grace of the Ascended Masters and the skill of a spiritual teacher are required for the skillful means to cut through all of the obstacles we create. Yet most, through ignorance, belittle the power of a teacher into the personality and cannot connect with the Ascended Masters in a pure way, beyond the filters of ignorance. Through the activations obtained within Eternal Yoga, we can better sift nectar from the inseparable quicksand of unconscious creation and understand the divinity of a teacher, all of creation, and most importantly—ourselves.

Eternal Yoga gives us a view. There is still much to do, but at least we now have the perspective and we can taste victory.

ETERNAL YOGA

Is

first achieving your victory within the Light

and

then the constant application of that victory into

full manifestation of the physically Ascended body

and consciousness.

Contents

1 Source of Teachings and Transmission 1

2 Key Understandings and Terminology 9

3 Initiatory Techniques of Eternal Yoga 35

4 Reality of the Higher Realms 61

5 Developing a Body of Light 75

6 Soul Development through the Rays of Light 115

7 Establishing a Retreat 179

Appendix 195

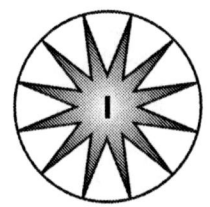

Source of Teachings and Transmissions

An Ascended Master coined *Eternal Yoga* in 1994, as Whitecloud and myself were finishing a retreat in the Himalayas, as to what we were to teach. Eternal Yoga originated entirely through inner transmission and direct teachings under various Ascended Masters. These understandings have occurred over many years and have become heightened through (and often originated because of) the coming together with my Twin Ray (Whitecloud AKA Shantara). To read more on the dynamics of the Twin Ray, see the companion books and our web site as listed in the appendix.

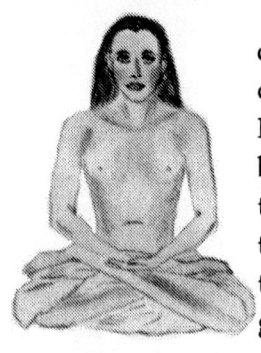

Many of these transmissions and the day-to-day guidance and refinements have come from my principal guide and root-guru, Mahavatar BabaJi, who maintained a physical body for over 2200 plus years. In the Tibetan tradition, he is Padmasambhava, having come to Tibet from India in the eighth century. Every teaching, every teacher, every consort, every grace, and the very emptiness, I either instantly or at some point experience as originating out of Mahavatar BabaJi. This is not poetical praise or something I have to work at realizing or some technique. For me, it is simply the way it is, and I feel very honored and blessed to experience it. Literally, without Mahavatar, I do not exist; a few times, he has literally maintained this body through actual death.

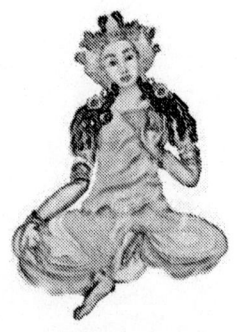

His Twin Ray and principle consort, Tara, has also been very active in giving me the tantric initiations and helping me with the refinements. Tara has helped to open within me the inner space in which to feel the Body of the One and through love, gain confidence in this love. To feel Tara simultaneously in a pool of water, in the trees, in the air, inside my chest in ecstatic happiness—to feel Tara as Love—to see her in many forms and to see Tara herself, is her grace. Tara first asked me to write these tantras into words and, in a dream, gave me a golden pen to do so.

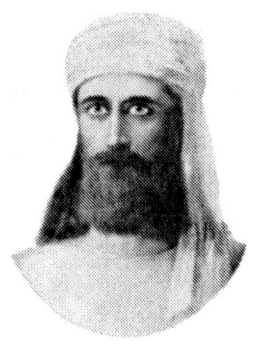
The Ascended Master El Morya (who through his kindness brought us into close retreat with him) is also inseparable from the concept of a root-guru for me. He has helped me beyond measure and it is by his grace that I have a heart by which to serve. The loyalty and love within his school is eternal and everflowing. I received the name Virochana from El Morya, who had previously carried that name. It was under El Morya, in retreat in the Himalayas, that we gained great insight into the depths of Eternal Yoga. It is by El Morya's blessings and urgings that this particular book has come into being and that Eternal Yoga is taught. He is exemplary of the purity of looking to spirit, by which we achieve fruitful results.

The Ascended Lady Master Leto continues to broaden my potential of tantra and the understanding of integrating the buddhic and physical realms. Having created a tantric body of nectar, she is a very amazing and skillful being, for whom this earth has much to be grateful. It was her Twin Ray, Gaylord, who coined the term, "Eternal Yoga." Gaylord is a Master of service towards a better world.

The Ascended Masters Meru and Aramu are parents of awesome beauty, care, and wisdom who bring special qualities of fluidity and cosmic empowerment within the tantric path benefiting countless beings. VajraYogini and Sita are other forms of Aramu. Meru is also known as Garab Dorje, Rama, an ancient founder of the Bon School in Tibet, and a leader and mystic 2400 years ago in North America. It is because of Meru 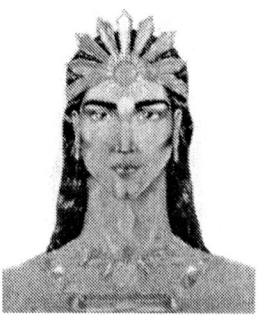 and Aramu that the highest tantric schools will reawaken and advance through these times. They are cosmic Masters of indescribably skillful means, fully empowered to use the cosmic override through eons of service. I have witnessed Meru moving the stars of destiny in the nighttime sky as easy as the movement of a hand. The love and blessings of Meru are incredibly tangible, guiding us in small and large details.

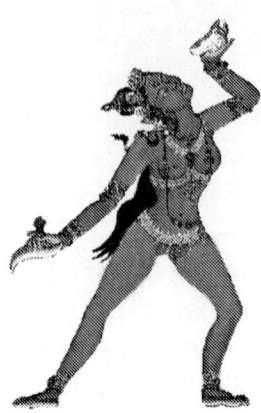

Meru and Aramu are the overseeing principle of the cosmic Mandala of Ascended Masters dedicated to the welfare of our earth. This Mandala of Masters will continue to bring this planet through the ravages of the destructive tendencies upon her. There is a saying about Meru and Aramu sung by the angels amidst ecstatic music, "They said it could not be done, but they have done it."

VajraYogini is the very construction of the universe itself: nectar, kindness, intimacy, passion and light—and very straightforward. Thus, she helps me to know the nature of existence—visibly and ecstatically indivisible. By being herself, Aramu has returned me to myself. For many she is the Earth Mother, in the sense that there are certain doorways and advancements connected with having a body that can only occur on this earth through her permission and grace. For those who have abused these teachings, her grace is their needed salvation.

I am especially grateful to Meru in his form as Garab Dorje for his kindness in giving me direct understandings of how to apply the tantras to achieve the Great Perfection and indestructible body. This transmission is included in the book, *Tantra as a Complete Path* (see appendix). Similarly, the whole family of Masters who have achieved the eternal body of light through the Great Perfection, including those listed above and many more, are inseparable from this Body of the One and thus also give their transmissions of love and inseparable wisdom. As in the words of Yaheshawa (Jesus), *"We serve the One, We are the One, We live for the One. No part is complete without the Whole."*

I would like to thank the Karamapa for his timeless transmissions, mostly under the form of the 16th Karamapa. He is one of the few 12th level adepts on the planet. Dilgo Kyhentse blessed me to create Books of Light Publishing. I wondered why a practitioner of his status did not create the eternal body in the present life, as he certainly had the ability to finish the

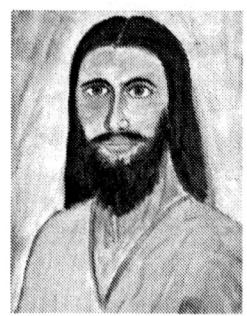
application. He told me that he has two more lifetimes. In his answer I better understood how in the enlightened view, ascension is not something for individual benefit or desired through ambition; in the bliss of our soul, we create a current that involves others in the big picture—for ascension occurs in the Body of the One.

There are many more Masters and practitioners of the path who have helped me greatly, including Koothumi and Saint Claire, Saint Germain and Lady Nada, the Master Ariel, Lantro and WindSong. I can go on and on, and each is priceless beyond description.

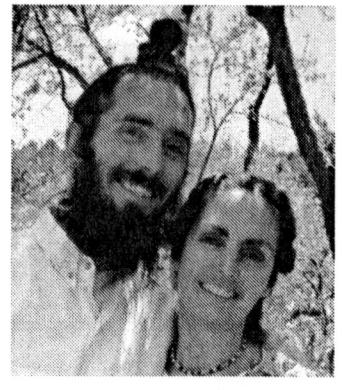

The framework in which I learned these tantras developed under the dynamics of the Twin Ray. This relationship has created a mutual way of seeing and overcoming subtle obstacles, transforming these very obstacles into expanding horizons, and has presented the inescapable checks needed to reveal and counteract spiritual ambition. These are normally the dynamics expressed in a teacher-student relationship, yet having these dynamics under the mutually equal and empowered Twin Ray relationship has allowed the limitations of a dharmic-based teacher-student role to be bypassed long enough for self-definition to establish awareness in the continuum of a greater existence.

Because of the physical reality of the Twin Ray, our teachers could exist primarily in a subtle embodiment.[1] Subtle and blissful dynamics extending into the buddhic realms can bind our soul in

---

[1] Note that I mention, "Primarily subtle embodiment." A number of the Masters have appeared into the physical for us at key moments and will do so in the future. This school works from the inside out, from the subtlest levels outward. These are actual beings that have applied themselves through the eons in their service towards Mastery. There is a very definite lineage of Masters.

god-realms for eons. It is the point of wisdom from the purity of spirit that penetrates through and within the desire body[2] to keep it on track and thus allowing the tantras to bear fruit in terms of ultimate liberation and integration. This is a gift of the Twin Ray. Some teachings openly state that only the Twin Ray can wield the cosmic rays correctly.

In stating gratitude to the Masters, it all comes to the Body of the One. What can be said of one particular Master can be said of many. The love of Tara is also Meru. The strength of Mahavatar is also El Morya. A Master is a Master to every other Master, and the quality an Ascended Master brings into universal beingness is available through all the Masters. The form is fluid, the consciousness is fluid, the moment is exact, the self is known and it is the Body of the One.

I pray that this and our other books will principally help the struggling western concepts of tantra and the tantra of Ascension. While the reality principles of the higher tantras, i.e., Ascension, are unchanging, the ways are countless. Thus the Americas, just like India, Tibet and China have previously done, will again develop their own approach.[3]

---

[2] While from a common perspective the desire body is simply the collection of our wants and preferences, in the tantric language, the desire body has a special meaning. The desire body, in this usage, is our activity through bliss, particularly our activated presence of soul, the sambhogakaya body. In tantric practice, the tremendous bliss experienced is the activity of the desire body, the nectars of light, within it.

[3] Of course, there are ancient wisdoms already present in the Americas. However, to modern culture, much of this wisdom has been lost with only a shadow left in shamanistic traditions that fascinate outer seekers. Fueling much of the spiritual light in the Americas are the timeless qualifications and memories within the earth of the native Masters. Thus, there will continue to come forth Masteries of the highest levels from the original Americans. In the future, they will be restored much of their rightful dignity within their own land. Indeed, many of these Masters, invisible to ignorant eyes, are active now.

Source of Teachings and Transmissions

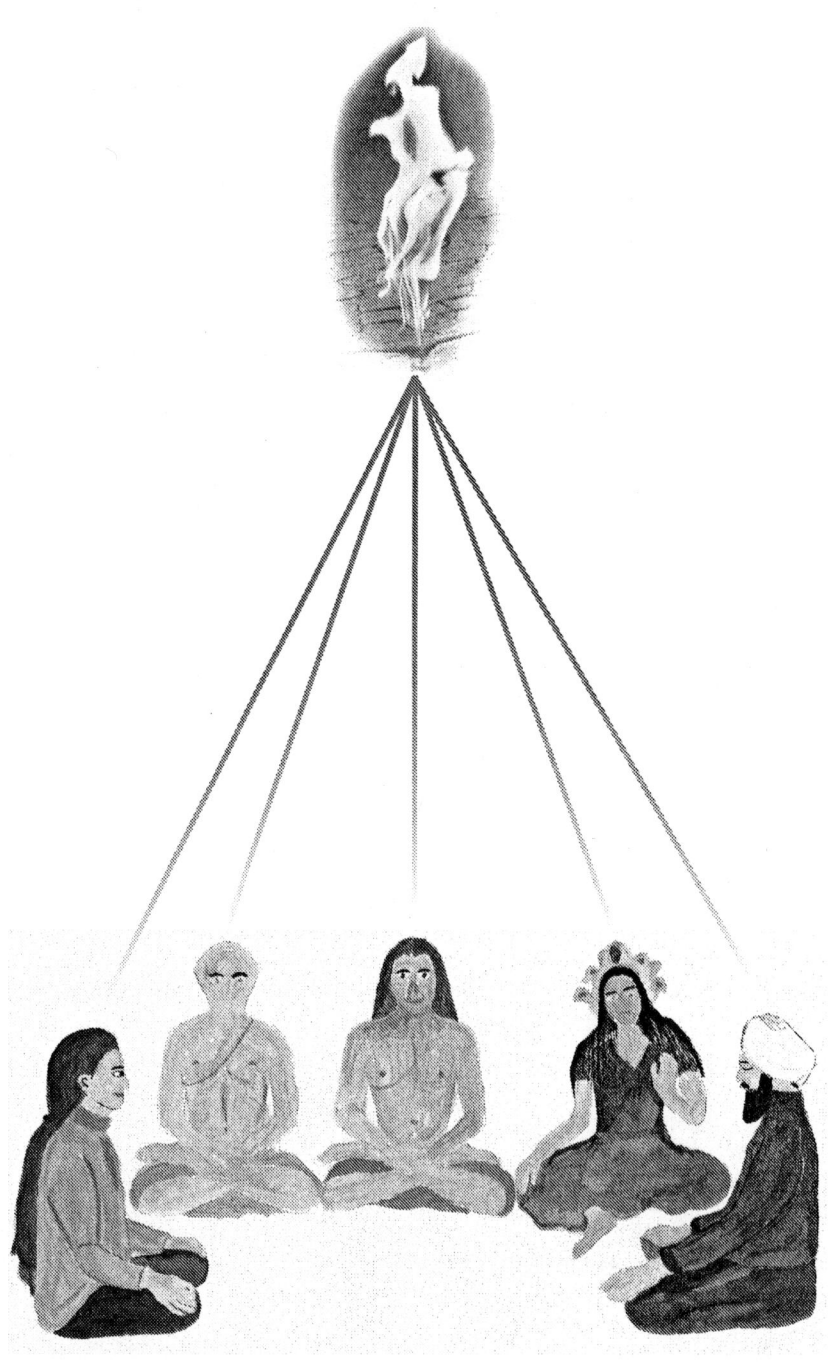

Key Understandings and Terminology

Presented here are key concepts, terms, and understandings common to this series of books. I recommended that you read this chapter several times.

Cultivating a Body of Nectar

Without bliss, the path is dry and filled with pursuits and doubts of the mind. Without bliss, experience comes and goes, yet nothing much changes. Bliss is timeless, it reveals our true nature, it consumes and creates—bliss is fuel for the spiritual path.

In a couple of classes, as we began, I asked, "Who has experienced real, mind-blowing, full-of-light, consuming bliss?" Many of these people have been on the spiritual path for more than a decade, and to my surprise, each time only one or two raised their hands, and often with some deliberation.

Spirituality, the art of knowing our spirit, is a very blissful affair. Nectar is our essence that makes spirit knowable in form and creating a body of nectar is a science that any of us can do. The first book of this series, *Cultivating a Body of Nectar,* gives methods to create enough clarity and vitality to cultivate the nectars of bliss.

Bliss consumes dogma, religion, prejudices, and fantasies. It lifts us naked and, in silent depth, it implodes and explodes. Bliss can hold the straightest face, walk the cleanest line, be the most grounded and make the most sense. In happiness, tranquility, compassion, even sadness and anger, a blissful being, always forgetting, never forgets who they are, because it is our nature lied bare and beautiful.

The spiritual path we present is not about instant fixes; rather it is for creating a foundation by which we can achieve lasting results. A body of nectar is cultivated, not instantly made manifest through fantasy and wishing. Through this body of nectar, we are fit to obtain all of who we are, for we have a body that can be it all. Let us start...

The Preliminaries of Yogic Development

Preliminaries focus on grounding, connectivity and presence through the yogic path of self-development. There are many methods and much skillful wisdom for this purpose. With this foundation, we can reach for the sky with our feet in spirit-nectar.

Practicing techniques without integration into our everyday life only gets us so far—and, why not adjust our lifestyle to create an atmosphere of discovery and richness? Areas of relationship, emotion, sexuality, self-responsibility, motivation, morality, diet, attitude, what we do for work and environment, are all a vital part of self-development. There is not so much a formula; rather, an obviousness of approach and emotional richness that becomes apparent as we continue. The details are usually somewhat different for each of us and different at various times in our lives.

There is a saying, "More practice, less drama. Less practice, more drama." The movement of energy and deepening awareness that occurs through yogic practice clears away much of the toxic and neurotic aspects of our life. We become centered in our peace and being. In the first few years of practice, it is necessary to be more interested in the radiance of our being than in the endless content of our emotions. Then, and only then, can we really listen to what our emotions are saying to us, from a soul perspective, and thereby use the energy of emotion as an integrated and necessary part of our enlightened clarity.

Yogic development revolves around a combination of passive and active practices. A kriya is an active practice that often uses a combination of breath (subtle and physical), visualization, mantra, posture, and even dynamic movement to create and deepen a nonverbal presence, which in turn supports meditative strengthening, deepening and discovery. In short, kriyas help to clear agitation, introduce us to the potential of our body and mind, and make us fit enough to apply ourselves one-pointedly.

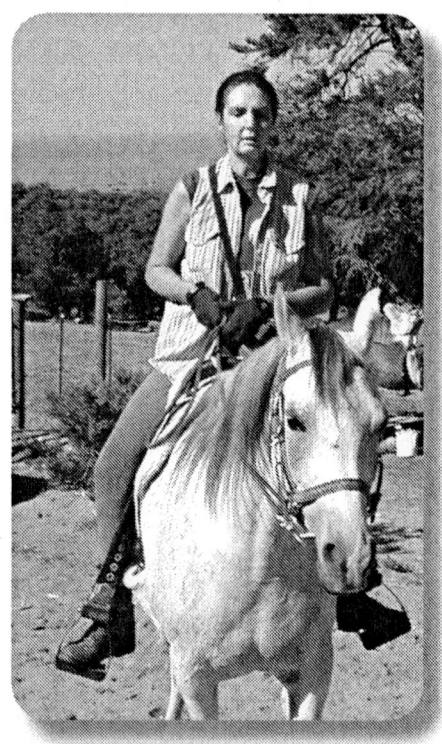

Passive practice is giving up into the surrender that realization is more than a technique. It is meditating through the natural wisdom of open awareness. Passive meditation is possible when the agitation of the mind cannot pull you in a million different directions, because the inner space is much more seductive, natural, alive, and vast than the quibbling and apparent force of the outer mind. There is not so much any one technique as a readiness for it. A typical example is still, silent, non-eventful meditation. At first, most people will have to move through agitation, and then boredom. If you can simply remain with and inside yourself, after a while your radiance will peek through the boredom. It is inevitable, because there is nothing else going on. Your life force is becoming one-pointed in its own natural intrinsic quality of bliss, and this bliss, when truly known, holds a much greater attraction for the outer mind than anything does of the world. If anything else is going on, you give up on it, not because you have to, but because you want to (although at first, you give up on it through faith in the practice). When you really give up, not like a depression, but in a way of letting go of anything or anyone or even your own idea of self, you relax into a radiant-emptiness. There is an inner sense of space. It is a very open feeling, which in time develops into a true awareness—where our innermost sense of effortlessness, aliveness, and natural awareness, is a continuum into everything that is. We experience this continuum simply through resting in the non-dualistic nature of our inner aliveness, not through effort.

Refined spiritual sensations and experiences need to have a space in which to occur. This is why we create the sense of space inside of us. Without this openness, it is difficult to trust that the spiritual path has more validity than the struggle. We simply give up on our intellect, our grasping, and our pride as anything that is going to get us anywhere. This openness, the experience of radiant-emptiness, is the only way to move past doubt.

Kriyas will open up an inner space, which will give you an initial feeling of the oneness of existence (the one flavor). Nevertheless, it is transitory. Through the passive practices, you discover it independent of props. A person can do many techniques, but they just become part of the wheel of endless experience until a person gives up on the wheel. When a person is willing to apply this aspect of the path, then they are truly ready. Everything else is secondary: work, happiness, accomplishment, bliss, our personality, everything is the scenery. Later, we reintegrate with the scenery in a very spectacular way. However, if we try to do it from an egotistical sense, it becomes just another egotistical extension.

Passive practices are not appropriate in the beginning; rather, one has to become ripe for it. You have to have had enough experience to know that there is something more. The active techniques get you clear enough so that you actually have the capacity to sit and ground within the vastness of inner space and discover something else. A core of prana is developed that can support an awareness that is rich and effortlessly nonverbal, and within that, you deepen into and relax within your true nature. A passive practice is not going for a walk or taking a nap. It is a very deep penetration of dissolving and then rediscovering ourselves. To really open up and let go requires a magnetic grounding inside of our bodies. To ground inside our bodies requires connectivity. Then we can let go from an inner core and the effect is total. Spacing out is not a very effective passive practice. This is not about dullness, sleepiness, or excitation; rather, a deeper presence that we are beyond grasping. It is often the first experience of unconditioned bliss, even if only a cozy bliss. **The two ways of practice, active and passive, work hand-in-hand.**

The working together of active and passive practice opens the tantric path. Through the specifics of particular techniques and the skill of relaxing our ego, we learn how to remain within our inner core. Within this originality of ourselves, we do not have to imagine or try to create emptiness and radiance, it is the original and natural condition. When we go to the ocean, we do not have to imagine what water looks like, because it is the scenery, it is the environment and, in this case, it is us.

Eternal Yoga

Eternal Yoga is a way of discovering our eternal nature. In this practice, we go above the head to aid this discovery. Through the success of Eternal Yoga, we will understand what our body, soul, and spirit is—beyond any doubt!

With this understanding, we can build upon our initial foundation to go all the way on the spiritual path, achieving liberation within eternal awareness. By bringing forth a bigger expanse, we have the opportunity for much greater self-definition. In radiant clarity, we will learn how to release the contraction of our individual grasping so that we gain freedom within our true nature.

Becoming aware of our continuum of spirit, soul, and body, we awaken the effortless light within. In silently acknowledging this, we enter into non-dual awareness. Awareness of this light is what makes possible further growth on the spiritual path. Through the activations of Eternal Yoga, we gain the ability to see and overcome our seed-karmas. The Blessing Presence so developed becomes the conduit of transmission and merit that makes our continued growth possible.[1]

During this time, we become aware of the Ascended Masters in a way that is not separate from us. Non-dualism becomes more than just a word as, "We get there by being there." Spirituality starts to warm up in a very special way. We begin to realize that enlightenment, ascension, and bodies of light are actual possibilities.

Transmission

Advancement along the paths of Eternal Yoga and tantra is dependent upon transmission. Transmission is a direct sharing that occurs within a common experience of Oneness. Even if words are involved, the essence of transmission is always non-verbal (not just an intellectual understanding).

The highest levels of transmission, the type we most care about in Eternal Yoga, come from entering into attunement with the Body of the One. As an example, to feel the presence of the Ascended Master El Morya is the transmission of his presence. From such a transmission, you can get a taste for and understand things that are impossible to explain in words alone. As an analogy, a happy person, simply by being who they are, tends to share, to give a transmission

---

[1] It is only through this awareness that the process of liberation can begin, in the context of liberation within a lifetime or two.

Key Understandings and Terminology 15

of their happiness to others. Therefore, even if you are not happy—by hanging out with a happy person, some of it might start to rub off on you. This is much more effective than reading about happiness in a book.

On the spiritual path, we use various skillful means to help create an atmosphere in which transmission can occur. For example, placing a picture of a loved one on your dresser helps you to feel that person, to connect with them. Likewise, we can use images of the Masters, sacred words, gratitude, and the cultivation of enlightened qualities, such as an open heart, to help prepare the space for connection and to facilitate the connection itself. Most importantly, clearing our mind of clutter and preparing the inner space allows us effortless connection in perfect timing.

While Eternal Yoga includes a cultivation of atmosphere and refinement into sacred space, concerning the actual moments of realization, it is instantaneous. Eternal Yoga emphasizes direct penetration into our own nature as the primary means of entering the sacred space in which instantaneous realization (transmission) occurs. This is at the heart of these teachings. Direct penetration is not a roundabout affair, nor an analytical process; rather, it is simply dropping the outer play of the mind and going straight to the essence. It uses skilful means to facilitate this non-dualistic state.

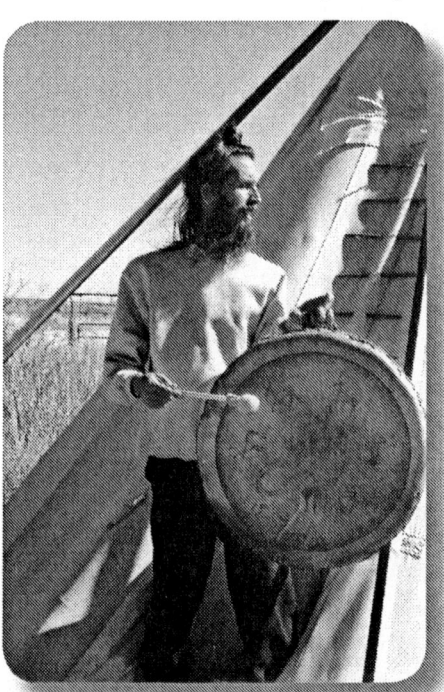

To illustrate what this means, consider two different ways of connecting to the Ascended Master Padmasambhava. You could buy a Tibetan tanka painting and read some books about this Incredibly Great Master. Then you could visualize the tanka painting everyday. You could visualize yourself looking exactly like Padmasambhava and imagine yourself doing all the things he did. You could also visualize all his companions surrounding you, being sure to get every color, detail, expression correct according to what you have read. The idea is that eventually, through this cultivation of sacred space, we might actually connect to this Master and through transforming ourselves into his image, obtain enlightenment. This is a possibility.

In Eternal Yoga practice, we take a different approach. To attune to a Master, there is no need for elaborate visualization. We simply attune to the presence, in the same way you would become aware of the presence of your spouse or loved one. We let the ever-changing details naturally fill in through direct awareness. For some, the question arises, "How do we attune to a Master if we do not know the feeling, the presence. How do we start?"

We can use some of the elements of the first approach to help create sacred space; however, this is a secondary, not a primary approach. To attune to a Master, we first attune to ourselves and deepen our awareness within the space of Oneness. We lift our consciousness and transform our own image. We examine our own nature. We practice continually returning to our own presence beyond the need to grasp at it. In this direct approach, nothing remains hidden. We honestly earn what we achieve. Along the way, we may remember the feeling of Padmasambhava from a past connection, or feel it from another who has had that connection, or simply the Master noticing you as you are ready. It is an honest connection, either it is there or it is not. We do not grasp at it. We also recognize that whenever we think of someone, even hear that person's name, on some level we have a connection. We cultivate the space of this awareness in the purity of our own being. There is aliveness on our side that meets an aliveness of another. Through gaining subtle awareness, we become aware of our subtle connections. It is instantaneous and effortless, not contrived. The work is simply preparing the grounds of our own being, and then we participate in the universe and meet other beings who are also participating in a similar manner. This is the family of the Masters, all living in the Body of the One.

Tantra

While the popular understanding in America of the word tantra is about sex, a truer understanding is, "Development of a refined energy body directly aware of itself originating from source." As a path, tantra starts with development of the Inner Temple and concerns itself with the continuum and the continuity of conscious presence. Tantric practice, at times, works with passion and blending; thus, sexual union is an invaluable aspect, provided the ability and awareness of working with refined energy is already present.

Tantra is awakening from our inner depth—outwards. Mistakenly, many try to go about this from the other direction, and simply go in circles.[2] When we are ready, Eternal Yoga practices give us the inner awareness necessary for tantric cultivation.

The book, *Tantra as a Complete Path (see appendix)*, gives wisdom and a few practical methods of further awakening within this core. As we advance, we are able to use our desires, passions and characteristics as the basic energy to enlighten all the ins and outs of our existence. It begins by sharpening the vision gained in Eternal Yoga, of making everything appear more transparent or less solid, and as the outer skin of an underlying divinity. In doing so, we ignite an inner core of presence within our body, and through further skillful application, we create an Inner Temple from which our appearance radiates forth. The possibility of bringing forth an Eternal Body of consciousness presents itself within this development of the nectar body.

Tantra is a path of a thousand corrections along the way. If you have a rigid disposition, are tightly bound in social consciousness, or do not understand the how and why of various practices, then you will not intuitively be able to make these corrections. Sensitivity to these thousand plus corrections requires that we listen, and it is one of the reasons that an experienced teacher is necessary. A skillful teacher helps us to hear what we are listening for—and in

---

[2] Working from the outside in is the subject of the preliminary yogas, lifestyle adjustments, replacing negative thoughts with positive thoughts, etc.—not the tantras. The yogas and similar approaches are much more effective and giving of fruit for this stage of practice.

the process, returns us to our self. A few advanced souls can get this feedback through subtle interaction with a teacher, but most require a physical interaction.

Tantra is a path of intensity and transformation, where we intensify our passions while bringing them into the emptiness of our Inner Temple. This is another way of saying that we find ourselves in essence beyond personality and beyond our individuality. The bliss within that indivisible union of outer and inner further reveals the perfection that underlies everything. We let go, while simultaneously radiating profound existence in all its varied peculiarities and plays.

Because there is so much transformation that occurs within the tantric path, some teachers mistakenly characterize tantra as a path of transformation. From a soul perspective, real transformation is not possible until we experience a profound peace with everything exactly as it is.

The transformative aspect of tantra becomes possible, from "a tantric perspective," only after we are beyond the dualistic views often associated with transformation itself. Then we are truly in the experience of ever-expanding perfection. Applying concepts of tantra, no matter how skilled our application, without a non-dualistic awakening, is not tantra. Even if the experience is wonderful, without an enlightened framework, it is like rising up on a swell in an endless ocean of experience.[3] Some will say it makes no difference what you call it; they feel a lot of happiness and growth in their so-called tantric lifestyle.[4]

---

[3] Of course, transformational activity can be and is beneficial, in regards to the spiritual path. This is one of the functions of kriya and purification. While very important and it helps to prepare the way, nevertheless, it is not enough in itself.

[4] This is not to devalue what people experience, and the lightness they find in liberating their energy into a more heart-felt expression. However, how far does it take you? Understand the power of illusion, for there is nothing else in all of existence, manifest for you to see and experience. Through the desire body reigning as king and queen, the path of tantra becomes a free-for-all, which has little to do with how it is taught and experienced by the Masters who have used it to get where they are. In stating these misconceptions of what the tantric path truly is, I am attempting to raise it back up in the minds and hearts of my students and readers, to its full glory.

What makes what I am saying even harder to comprehend are convincing moments, such as, "If the beauty of sexual union is not non-dualistic, then what is?" This distinction is nevertheless important to understand because one application leads nowhere, in terms of spiritual liberation, and the other is an enlightened application into liberation. You get there be being there. Tantra requires an activated awareness within the buddhic realms and beyond. You must know this beyond doubt, there can be no question about it. You need to understand the relationship of spirit into soul into physicality in the full sacredness, beyond personality. The trapping is that without this, we are spellbound within our personality, for we do not know anything else. Even if we briefly experience the purity of direct connection, without recognizing it and gaining familiarity, we forget it. We are simply rising up and down on the endless swells of our limited perceptions, i.e., the endless cycles of death and rebirth, our world.

The Great Perfection

The Great Perfection is an enlightened view, not a technique. Through deepening, transmission, and surrender, we taste the Great Perfection and then diligently blossom this awareness into fruition.

Your heart literally sings a song of indescribable beauty, manifesting as creation itself. Within you is a pinpoint of eternal depth that at any and every moment is everything. You, me, the room you are in, and the book you are reading is all the same space and everything within this is simply as it is. The mind is space, love is space, space is nectar and through the nectars of space in the bliss of the One, we have creation. We are here—ignorant or not, in hell or heaven—perfection underlies appearances of stench and perfume alike.

The Great Perfection is being in non-dual awareness. Entering into the Great Perfection is the fruit of Eternal Yoga. The Great Perfection is remaining in the underlying reality of spirit throughout the continuum of manifestation.

Non-dual awareness, when used as the underlying empowerment of a practice, such as the tantras, has several themes:

- *Getting there by being there.*

- *Knowing how to get out of your own way.*

- *An underlying effortlessness of awareness.*

- *Effortlessly knowing how to use space as a support for consciousness.*

- *Awareness of all of this within your heart.*

The Great Perfection is the beginning, the application, and the fullness of a liberated being. The Great Perfection is how we see and experience everything through enlightened perception. It is the ultimate attitude, effortlessly given, containing within it a thread supporting a continuation of enlightened existence.

Eternal Yoga helps us to enter into awareness of the Great Perfection from the level of higher mind. However, as wonderful as this is, we still must bring forth the completeness of this view into our everyday life. This is tantra. Eternal Yoga is the aspect of tantra that introduces and emphasizes the proper perspective whereby the tantric path may bear fruit.

Not everyone chooses to extend this view into everyday life. Some, who have the karmic purity to allow it, choose to withdraw solely within the buddhic light of the Great Perfection. The sole object of cultivation is remaining within the rarified atmosphere of the buddhic realms. While skillful means can be used to more quickly see the buddhic light within our everyday experience, the resulting vision is used for further withdrawal into the soul realms. There is nothing else to do, other than remain in this awareness. All of this, it should be emphasized, has the special awareness of the buddhic realms themselves as a quality of spirit. There is no emphasis to understand oneself in terms of the details of relationship, awareness within the earth, or within all the ins and outs of our world. As the soul withdraws, this often results in a gradual disappearance from the physical world altogether.

Such a practitioner has remained steadfastly and solely within the rarified vision of the Path of the Great Perfection, seeing nothing else, and if successful in remaining centered within spirit (what the Buddhist call dharmakaya), reaps liberation into these soul realms (what the Buddhists call sambhogakaya). That means they are an active presence within these realms able to benefit all who attune to them in that capacity—a very high achievement indeed.

It is important to remember, that as we truly enter into this state of consciousness, the importance we give to our immediate personality and its ambitions diminishes, and as such, we are transparent to a much greater activity, inherently understood within the perfection itself. The feminine has come into play. This activity, while we may steadfastly start out within one approach or another, may precipitate a change of plans, so to speak.

Broadening this view through the skillful application of the nectars within our body to embody awareness of and within the Body of the One, results in an active divine consciousness within the world. This is the tantric path. In the tantric path, we appear to embrace separation and see the value of separation itself as part of the perfection. It is a dance. Of course, this is dynamic, at times appearing totally to withdraw, and at other times, actively embracing the same light within our everyday lives. There seldom is a one or the other approach, and there is no black and white dividing line.

In the United States, the Great Perfection was presented through a profound, yet seldom-understood and mostly misrepresented approach called the "I Am." The I Am teachings of Saint Germain are a very simple, direct and, at the same time, an extremely advanced approach. Unfortunately, most use the teachings as an extension of the ego—I Am, rather than a true awakening within the Body of the One. It requires a lot of deepening to properly receive and apply these transmissions.

Masters of the Dzogchen teachings of Tibetan Buddhism and the Bon Dharma present the Great Perfection as a path along with the underlying transmissions. This is a rich and potent lineage of transmission.

Eternal Yoga, Dzogchen, and the I Am teachings, while using different methods, all have the same underlying aim, to introduce you to direct awareness of yourself and your perceptions as spirit. In fact, all three of these approaches have the same lineage of Masters.[5] Whatever terminology is used: God, enlightenment, the dharmakaya, or spirit—the direct introduction itself is beyond dualistic understandings of any terminology. Any method with this aim will always emphasize the importance of its Masters, for the direct awareness introduced and the consciousness of the Masters is no different. The Masters are the means, i.e., the active principle, by which this transmission occurs. All of the skillful means of these paths are simply ways to refine your awareness and to get you to notice.

Some ignorant teachers present the idea that you first progress through the tantras to get to the place where you are ready for these teachings. This has created a lot of confusion as to what the tantric path is, isolating it as transformative techniques of a dualistic nature, essentially treating the tantras like kriyas.[6]

When teachings of tantra and the Great Perfection enter into a religious structure or mass teaching, this type of distortion is inevitable (by trying to fit the tantric path within a social framework, when it cannot be so tightly contained). The work of the Great Masters, while being of enormous service to many, has always been to bring in one person at a time. As far as the inner teachings are concerned, there is no such thing as a mass teaching.

In truth, to enter the tantras, you must first taste the Great Perfection. Without a non-dualistic view from which to apply the tantras, you will only be working with a set of techniques. Developing a yogic foundation gives us enough clarity and non-verbal awareness

---

[5] Respectively: Padmasambhava, Garab Dorje, Saint Germain. These are the principal masters recognized as the fathers of these lineages, although of course, there is a whole body of recognized and unrecognized Masters behind each lineage. Within all of these lineages, the same family of Masters is at play.

[6] This comment is particularly addressing the way Dzogchen is commonly presented in relation to the Tibetan tantras. In the institutionalized presentation of the Tibetan tantras to the west, there is often lacking the small, family-like atmosphere in which the Master teaches. Often ignored is the requirement of years of discipline. Thus, trying to keep things sacred, yet not receiving the heart application, we end up putting ourselves into a spell, or else lose the sacredness required. Through the foundations and atmosphere of intimacy with enlightened beings, we relax into the non-dual awareness necessary to begin the practices, and inwardly receive the true, ongoing teachings.

to practice the techniques of Eternal Yoga. Through the insights and refinement thus gained, we become ready to enter the tantric path.

Both tantra and the pure Great Perfection paths have the same empowering truth—both are cultivations of non-dual awareness. Further journeying on the tantric path develops skillful means, giving us an ability to benefit more people. Tantra uses skillful means and transformation to recognize the Body of the One, and thus broaden our view of the Great Perfection. This broadening eventually results in the penetration of a Body of Light all the way into the physical.

The Great Perfection approach uses pure awareness and its inherent energy as the path itself, awakening within and as the light of the soul. Every thought you think and every emotion you feel is experienced as originating from an efflorescent place of spirit. The play of creation may end up qualifying the formless radiance of energy into a thought such as "yuck." Within pure awareness, we remain conscious of the underlying source radiance, spirit, prior to its eventual qualification. This source radiance has within it the infinitely responsive and inherent wisdom in how any stream of thought can be turned around back into a harmony with the entire universe, from the perspective of source. This brings forth another popular Dzogchen concept into play, "By remaining in pure awareness, thoughts (and scenarios) self-liberate into the highest possible outcome." Insignificant thoughts simply dissolve, as there is no better purpose for them, and through it all, you get to enjoy the radiance of spirit itself. There is no way you can lose. There is nothing to embrace, no vows to keep, nothing to transform, just pure awareness revealing itself. There is a popular Dzogchen saying, "The sickness of effort has been overcome."

The emphasis might be on the purity of the Great Perfection or the skillful embrace of the Tantras, depending on the disposition and perfection of the moment—inwardly they are not separate.

In a sense, even a pure Great Perfection path is also tantric in nature, for by advancing upon it, we become intimate with the underlying elemental light-play of form and formlessness. Because the practitioner has learned unwaveringly to remain aware, this transmission of the light-play remains ever-present; lifting, connecting, deepening, and absorbing our everyday awareness into the power and presence inherent within it.

Even the phase, "The Great Perfection," denotes a tantric embrace of the world through the enlightened state. To say that after tasting the Great Perfection, I will further advance on the tantric path, is another way of saying, "My heart is so opened up in the divine flow that it swells up in compassion, and soaked in this love, I skillfully apply my self, through the perfection of Divine mood, for the benefit of all beings." Tantra is experiencing oneself as an active exuberance of the divine, beyond the ability of a limited personality to say otherwise. You see all, even the most horrible disagreeable beings, or even beings who you must outwardly oppose, in essence, as light. This is the Great Perfection. Sitting down in a room, while others may experience nothing particular, you experience yourself floating in primordial space. You experience rocks levitating exactly where they are. It is just how it is.

The purity of the Great Perfection is not a puritanical purity, rather the efflorescence of spirit itself forever bubbling up within the heart and radiating with an invisible light. If you could see it as a physical light, it would appear to be made of a million suns. The inner landscape of the so-called pure path of Dzogchen looks very tantric at times, because it is far beyond the judgments of good and bad. The most advanced practitioners, because of their identity as spirit, can draw energy from chaotic environments that would deaden most practitioners. This is not a focus on transformation, but rather a grounding in source. The occasional adept that displays themselves through the crazy yogin or left-hand paths may actually be practicing more of a pure Dzogchen path than a tantric path.

To progress upon the path of Great Perfection requires an infinite ability of fluidity through grounding beyond the nature of outer realities, and its one absolute dependence is in bringing forth a relationship with a Master or Masters whereby the transmissions may occur in consciousness. In fact, it is impossible not to have a connection with a Master, for the heart of the Great Perfection is the Body of the One, which is composed of Masters, i.e., those who are awake. Without this, there is no heart; without the heart, there is no depth, and without depth, we are simply in a dualistic mind-set.

Dream Yoga

There are two aspects of dream yoga. One is cultivating the ability to dream with clarity and lucidity. In such dreams, we can do practice, project ourselves, gain understanding, perform service and transform the nature and content of our dreams.

A more advanced aspect of dream yoga is not about dreams at all, rather it is about absorbing our pranas within our central core and maintaining radiant, primal consciousness while we sleep. This is an aspect of tantric practice.

We all, regardless of spiritual practice or not, at times have pertinent and lucid dreams. However, dream yoga is experiencing this consistently.

Dream yoga is an incredible valuable part of practice. Success in this is a reflection of our daytime practice. Trying to gain mastery in this area without a strong daytime practice is extremely difficult, if not impossible. In times of intense practice, such as during a retreat, dream clarity and remaining awake within our core while asleep often occurs spontaneously and as a kind of after effect—a continuation of our daytime practice.

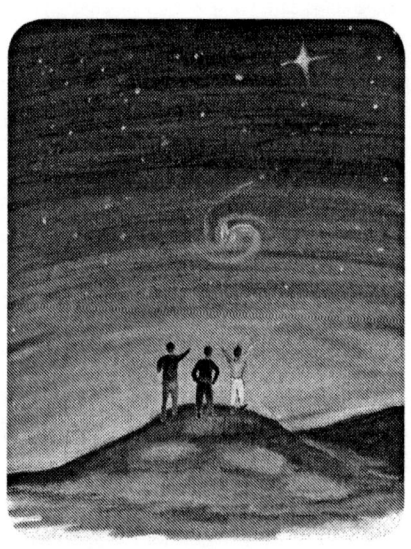

Motivation

Within our growth through these methods and transmissions is a concurrent refinement of our motivation, which is simply an opening of our heart. As we clean our own house, the ambition to achieve greater enlightened activity and presence changes from a self-centered activity to altruistic love and compassion. Far from the mushy heart, this is tremendous clarity born of and blended with wisdom beyond a conventional mind set. Consciously acknowledging the growing desire to benefit all beings ignites an even deeper outpouring of our heart. The radiance of this energy breaks through our contractions, by opening us to the enlightened nature in which it is born. We feel no great claim of being a Good Samaritan, for this compassion is merely reflective of the deeper nature of reality as oneness. An Ascended Body is none other than manifest radiance from within the Body of the One, displayed through you. The growing change of motivation within us is a clear sign as to our readiness to embrace the next stages.

Tantra blossoms into a free-flowing, blessing power through a heart-centered, good-natured, but not naïve attitude.

The tantric path is to be or to become a Blessing Presence.

Any other motivation plays havoc, because it is afraid of losing something called self.

Until a person is comfortable and clear in regards to relationship, sexuality, and intimacy, they are not yet ready for the tantric path. Being able to work with energy in a conscious, empowered and surrendered way (required in relationship) is part of this path.

A Teacher

In the more common spiritual paths, such as religion, the outer yogas, self-reflection, purification, etc., it is helpful but not necessary to have a teacher. However, as we fully enter the tantric path, a teacher or teachers are necessary for reasons of transmission and because we quickly enter into difficult areas of our psyche. The relationship with a teacher is very sacred. Only those people who live in sacredness can understand this relationship. The tantric path requires divine intimacy, respect, and wisdom with a teacher to facilitate the necessary ongoing transmission.

We learn something by first experiencing a feeling or a sense of it, and then embodying that feeling under our own image so it becomes a natural part of our being. This is the primary function of transmission, i.e., the direct sharing of divine experience, which is possible through oneness. This is how you get an initial feeling or sense.

Without transmission, there is no real clear understanding of where we are going. It is all just words. There are many scriptural accounts of how students have undergone years or decades of service, preparation, and growth to enter into a space where transmission can occur, and where they are consciously aware of the transmission. Once profound transmission is experienced, then it is only a matter of application and stabilization—for the result has already been attained on a seed level. We get there by being there. While I am talking about profound transmission, the many thousands of small transmissions, the nuances we pick up from enlightened company and communion, are a vital part of the spiritual path.

A teacher on the spiritual path is someone you have given authority to. Thus, this person can question you, provoke and stimulate you, and communicate to you in areas you may not otherwise allow. Obviously, this requires surrender. Confusion arises in some people because they equate surrender with giving away their power. However, real surrender is impossible in a framework of disempowerment or blind worship. Real surrender will not occur as long as the lower mind plays around in confusion and in a toxic way. You must still do the work. Thus, a real relationship with a teacher is a mature and advanced state of sensitive communion and responsiveness. The outer mind becomes still.

For most people tantra is about passion and blending. Emotion, feeling, and passion are, as we become clear, the voltage that makes all this possible. As this happens, our feeling-ability opens up an inner, all-pervading space, which is infinitely delicate and embracing. There is an inspiring beauty of using attachment, desire, intimacy and emotion to fuel our awakening within the natural state. Without a close relationship with someone who understands what we are being refined into, this process will become a circus and not yield the type of fruit that allows the work to begin on the Ascended Body within the space of one lifetime. A tantric teacher will use the power of emotion to bring forth definition within the emptiness, not within a mindset fixed on social conditioning.

The Twin Ray

In the light beyond the light, form beyond form, the Body of the One—from the perspective of the Individualized God-Self—the first outpouring into the manifestation is the Twin Ray.[7]

The Twin Ray is the root of all relationship, and as such, every relationship is ultimately only possible because of this initial outpouring.[8] While of Oneness, the universe is not vague. In our journey back into where we have always been, we can again come together with our other half in the physical, and thereby bridge all that lies between.

This greatly propels activation and awareness into the very subtle states that we are entering. Many look upon the Twin Ray as a romantic idea, and when they deeply fall in love with another, perhaps experiencing their relationship in a very subtle awareness, the thought occurs, "This person has to be my Twin Ray." That is, until likes and dislikes come into play, and then it was just a mistake.

The truth is that an awareness of the Twin Ray is impossible without buddhic awareness, and even with that, it still requires awareness beyond. Some think the Twin Ray is the same soul, this

---

[7] This is a very subtle outpouring; however, subtle is a relative term. From a physical perspective, the initial outpouring of the Twin Ray is extremely subtle. When you are not looking "at" the subtle realms with a consciousness conditioned from earthly perspective, but are totally within them, an idea can be more solid-like and tangible than a metal structure, or it can be just a wisp. The subtle outpouring of the Twin Ray into existence is the most definite structure existing in the entire universe, although it is solely consciousness.

[8] Do not think of this initial outpouring as a linear timing. It is a continual occurrence. By reawakening to this level, you are simultaneously at the beginning of and within time.

is not it. Each of us have our distinctly developed soul, or souls, for you can have more than one. All of this may be a bit mind-blowing, as it should be.

Once a master appeared to me in a subtle, yet physically visible form, and gave me the teaching, "You have three beloveds (Twin Rays)."

Your first Twin Ray is your Self. The only way towards becoming aware of your eternal partner is to first awaken within your self. Without this step, nothing is possible. The next Twin Ray is your eternal tantric partner. The third Twin Ray is the Ascended Body of the One.

Most people in their awareness are but small fragments of their soul, so in their current state, it is impossible to experience a Twin Ray relationship. If you want to move towards the Twin Ray, then you must first awaken within yourself. Awaken to and embody more of your soul. This is a gift of the spiritual path in general and Eternal Yoga specifically.

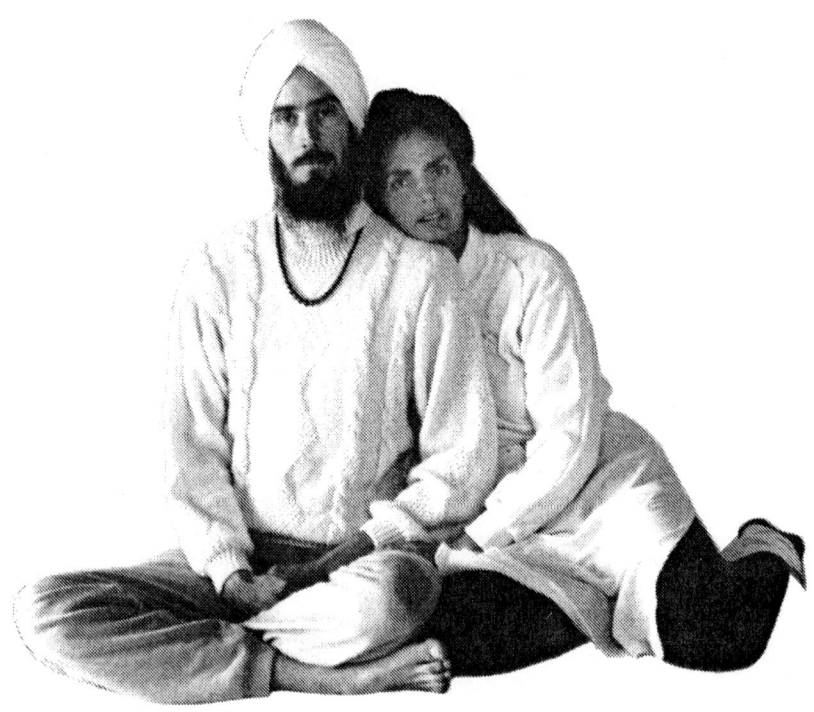

The Twin Ray relationship is, in essence, far beyond form. A partial energy of your Twin Ray can present itself through many people. One of the ways to move towards your Twin Ray is to treat every relationship with this intensity and sacredness. If you combine this with the unshakeable commitment to awaken within your self, then you will keep moving forward. When you embody enough of your soul into the physical, then that wholeness allows awareness of the truth of the Twin Ray to begin developing.

You only have one Twin Ray. It is not a choice, "I like this person and not that person; I think I will make this person my Twin Ray." The Twin Ray relationship can be very challenging, as everything you have ever experienced, from the level of buddhic outpouring down into all of your experience through the eons of incarnation, comes under its scrutiny. You have an authority with each other, that no other being has, not even the Ascended Masters. The Twin Ray is a tremendous potential to accelerate the alignment, into consciousness, of all you have ever been.

There are also traps within this relationship. Because of the tremendous intensity of what you elevate within yourself, the tremendous impact this has on many beings who you have woven within your lives through all time, and the closeness you have—it is easy to become attached. This can be appropriate, and somewhat unavoidable, for a time.

Looking to the form of the Twin Ray too much, rather than remaining connected in the essence of it, results in an impossibility of this light being brought fully into the physical, as required by the fullness of Ascension. Understanding that Ascension is a tantra, this is another way of stating a truth emphasized throughout this book, that tantra is not possible without the perspective of spirit. You have to have that view, and this view is not possible in attachment to form. The Twin Ray brings forth a very high level of Tantric application, one that cannot be done without the Twin Ray. This application includes a weaving of the universe itself, so if you are caught up in the personality, this weaving cannot occur. It is very challenging. The Tantra of the Twin Ray brings forth awareness of the Body of the One into its weaving of form.

You cannot fully ascend without the Twin Ray. If you are not conscious and embodying the root level of your manifestation, then there is no way you will bring that forth. At the same time, many Masters who are with their Twin Rays do not complete the Ascension, fully into the physical, because of the level of attachment. This results in the Ascension completed to the level of soul (Sambhogakaya realms), and requires further conventional rebirth for the opportunity to bring this down into the physical.

In her previous life, Whitecloud lived in a regenerating body, eternally youthful in appearance. This was in a cave with Mahavatar and other Masters. This body did not need to eat and was wonderful in many other ways. However, this was not enough; she needed to complete the tantric application with myself, her Twin Ray. We are aware of a number of other highly advanced Masters who are also incarnating at this time to complete this application.

The Twin Ray relationship helps you to see through distortions more easily. This is not a guarantee, you can also create distortions together, but when purely empowered, you have a way of seeing within the budhic realms from different perspectives that are shared from a root level. While this is not unique to the Twin Ray, it is most prevalent within this relationship. In short, you can see and move through obstructions and challenges much more quickly, making liberation within a single lifetime a possibility.

As a Twin Ray relationship awakens, it can only exist in a level of tremendous service. This is because the Twin Ray awareness, itself, originates within the domains of the bigger picture. As you progress, you move beyond the level of individuality, yet you remain an individual as well.

The tantric schools of the Ascended Masters are held from the level of the Twin Ray. The level of blending within these schools is very intimate. Each brings the transmission of another quality to another, and in this way, we expand. It can be very blissful. If the desire body becomes king, then a "pristine" awareness of spirit as source is lost. This is very subtle, and those who cannot continually make this distinction of source in the buddhic realms are simply not aware of it.[9]

---

[9] This is the classical blending of bliss and emptiness, of which the Buddhist tantras revolve around.

It is analogous to a very thin silk strand floating in the vastness of outer space. You may not even see it. In its authority into manifestation, this is the axis of what the Twin Ray revolves around. From the perspective of spirit itself, the difference of those who have this awareness and those who do not, is huge. It is the difference between, enjoying temporary life in the god realms, or true awakening within the Body of the One and thus Liberation within form.

Gaining awareness of the Twin Ray is an integral part of Eternal Yoga and the tantras. The book, *Tantra of the Beloved* (see appendix) has a chapter on the Twin Ray. The entire 600-page book revolves around this awareness.

Within these schools, there are those who, with an incomplete development, decided that they do not want any checks at all placed upon them. Tasting freedom through bliss, this is their truth. Yet, there is not the full understanding, and the paramount thread upon which success of the tantric path depends—unconditional and an unbreakable trust on a connection with an Ascended Master—was broken—traded for an illusion of self-grandeur in their play within the budhic realms. As the understanding of the Twin Ray was not yet fully realized, the teaching of the Twin Ray falls aside as well, as just another apparent blockage to their freedom of doing things exactly as seen fit.

Many of these personalities have continued in their incarnations bringing forth a distorted view of what tantra is. Some of these beings are beginning to realize that there is something more. This entire play, occurring through eons of times and involving seemingly countless incarnations, itself can be seen as an evolving activity, the Ever-Expanding Perfection. Ironically, the Twin Ray brings forth the greatest freedom imaginable—one that plays, yet is simultaneously beyond the play. It is through the authority of the Twin Ray that all is held in check and under the alignment of spirit. It takes a long evolvement in form, to come back within form with an awareness of where we eternally start from.

Once you perceive that silk thread emanating into creation from beyond, it is crystal-clear. This is not some law decided upon by the powers that be, but simply a reflection of creation itself. It is impossible to describe the fullness in words, not even a thousand volumes could do it, yet through direct experience, it is very obvious, profound, and simple. While we can take a long time to come into clarity, in many ways, clarity is the beginning of the path.

Ascension

Ascension is a western term for an aspect of the tantras where we transform our physical body into a body of light that remains active within the physical and subtle realms.

The ascension occurs through unveiling a way of seeing, whereby we experience everything as an elemental light quality—in totality. This vision[10] is not unique to the ascension; however, in the ascension, rather than dissolving the body into it, or losing awareness of the body altogether, we transform our body into a direct, active expression of this elemental mind.

There are various levels of mastery within the light body. For example, there are Masters who can temporarily project such a body as a penetration of their forever-existing extremely subtle body. There are those who effortlessly sustain it, those who can only sustain it within the consciousness of the earth and those who can sustain it anywhere in the universe. This body is not the same as ghostly apparitions or a temporary karmic projection from a being in god-like realms.

How regular, physical people perceive such a Master is a combination of a person's sensitivity, interior language, and a manipulation by the Master of the visual ability of others to perceive them. For example, there are yogis whom we have had contact with that are visible to some people and not to others.

A fully-developed body of light can only come about by the desire to benefit others; otherwise, because of self-absorption, it would not come about in its fullness. It is a gift from the Body of the One—for the Body of the One.

---

[10] This vision is more than sight. Sight is used for simplicity in trying to explain the unexplainable.

Love is

the Beginning

Middle

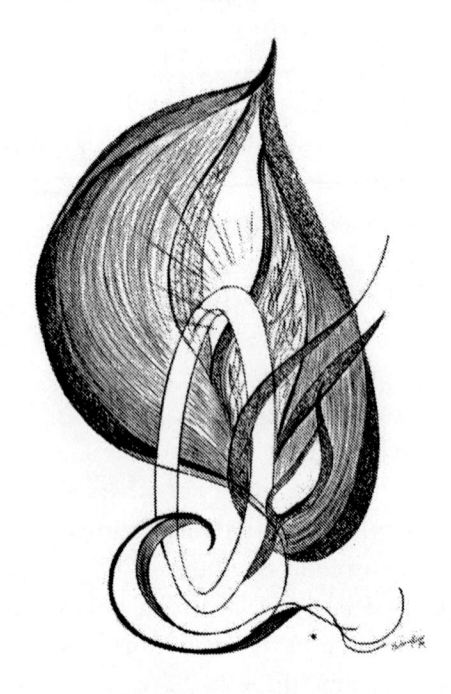

and End

INITIATORY TECHNIQUES OF ETERNAL YOGA

Regaining Awareness as a Body of Self-Generated, Effortlessly Radiant Light

The realization and acknowledgement that we are consciousness of unlimited potential, forever-radiating effortless light and form, containing Perfection at all times is the essence applied to bring forth our Ascension.

These meditations are profoundly simple, and for those who are not ready, easy to dismiss as ineffective. When you are ready for them, they are gold. In the awareness developed are the keys of awakening within buddhic awareness. Part of being ready is the ability to focus in a very subtle way beyond levels of psychic fascination and the grosser personality.

It is important to understand the difference between initiation and adeptship. Your mind is infinitely agile, it can tell you anything, show you any vision, lead you down any path and create all the confirmation or rejection that you desire. There is no way out but through. Often those who first touch into this subtlety of mind go down the garden path—being fascinated with the ease of phenomenal confirmation.

A competent guide can help us through the pitfalls and with our confidence. Keep the purity of your heart, remain humble, and continue moving forward. Mistakes can be our greatest teachers, if we have the humility to listen and the willingness to learn. If all we can do is think about ourselves or if there is a tendency to run after our mind, then it is better to focus on the foundational practices. Even when we are well settled, the Eternal Yoga practices are not a substitute for the power of simple kriyas to unite body, breath, and mind.

Read carefully, ask questions (my email address is in the appendix) and take the practices to heart everyday. These initiatory meditations are:

- *Creating the Inner Temple*
- *Connecting to Source*
- *Light Body Awareness*
- *I Am the Ever-Expanding Perfection*

In case this is not already crystal-clear—practice intensely to awaken in the subtle buddhic realms *only after* you have created an initial spiritual foundation. Otherwise, it is likely that you will simply manifest your grosser ego into subtle realms of ego and instead of liberation, will only further bind yourself in more subtle, and difficult to get out of, realms of delusion. I cannot emphasize enough how important a proper teacher is for guidance.

When you are ripe, it is as if you are hearing about and practicing what you already know, and it really feels right. You are not looking so much for an answer to your problems, rather, you want to be, and are, like lovers who do not need to say a word.

The other, more likely scenario, is that without preparation, nothing at all will occur, as the practitioner simply is not capable of holding such a refined focus long enough in the proper internal space. In this instance, the practitioner loses faith in the practices, because they have not experienced anything for themselves, thus creating obstacles to practice in the future. Techniques and wisdom to create a yogic foundation are presented in the books: *Tantra of the Beloved,* and *Cultivating a Body of Nectar: Kriya Yoga and Tantric Foundations* (see the Appendix.)

Some of us, because of work in previous lifetimes, will very quickly have experiences through Eternal Yoga practices as they consciously reconnect to their existing body of light. These souls will find the greatest attraction to these techniques. Most likely, this connection to their buddhic essence, their soul light, will already have occurred in various moments through this life. In this instance, upon a fuller activation, practitioners will quickly find themselves in the same position that they were in when they last consciously worked through this light. For example, if they previously did lots of wonderful activity through their subtle light body, this will come into play again. If they created for themselves subtle scenarios of resistance (ignorance) and un-enlightened dominion, this will come into play again.

It is not always easy to tell the difference between wonderful and deluded—and the undefined heart often does not care, not realizing its predicament. Until we establish an infallible connection to our underlying spirit, the currents of our fascinations, ambitions, blindness, and desires can easily sweep us away. A relationship with a teacher is about listening. In the proper alignment, there is no difference between the teacher and oneself. It is all telepathic. When for one reason or another, the alignment is not there, it is the physical words and actions of the teacher that is the lifeline. If you ignore that lifeline, you risk sinking into your own creations for however many eons it takes to figure it out.

Neither can a teacher do your path. A teacher cannot save you. A teacher cannot deliver you. There are no guarantees. Your teachers, when they find you and you find them, are like ropes of clarity to help you climb the mountain. A teacher is like a lover beyond words, but you must also be a lover. You must go through adolescence, willing to be clumsy, and keep moving forward in the love.

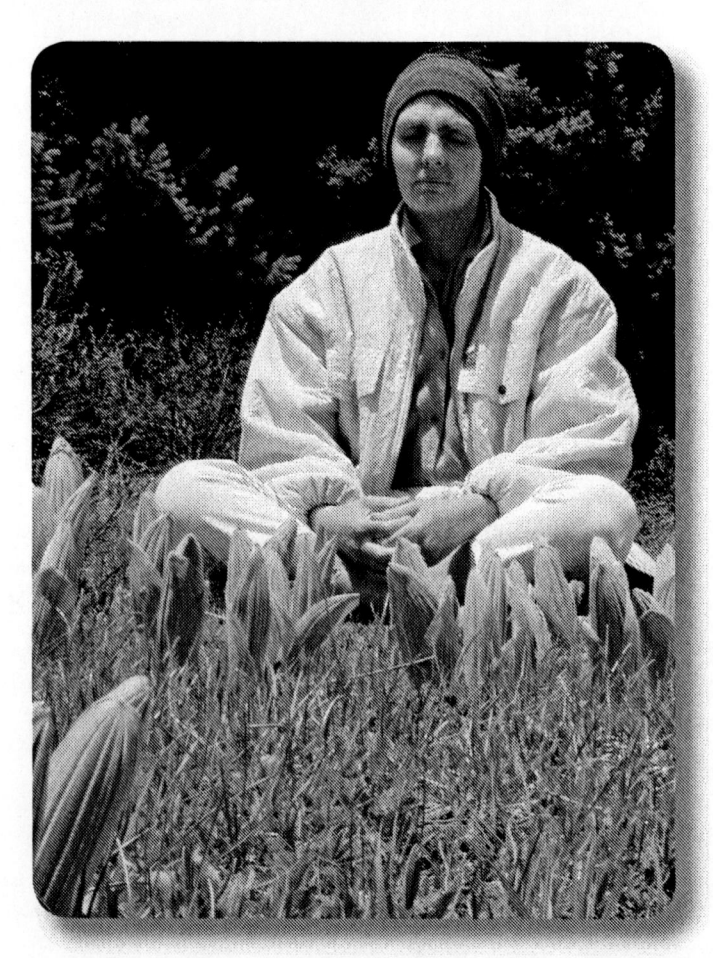

CREATING THE INNER TEMPLE

The Inner Temple is our innermost core of light and consciousness residing within our body. The fullness of this creation is an advanced tantric practice; however, we can begin the process now.

Through this visualization, we will refine our body enough so that it can anchor the energies we will use in the next practices. It is also very rejuvenating, playful, and enjoyable. You may substitute the warm-up exercises and visualizations with other practices of a similar nature; for example, yoga exercises of your own choosing and Taoist or Tibetan visualizations that work with the central channel.

The central channel is not the same as the physical spine, although it can overlap and reflect into the spinal marrow. While ideally we want to work with the deepest levels of the central channel, this is something that takes years to discover, thus it is permissible to work with the outer aspects, as long as the feeling is deep—as if your body could dissolve into and arise out of it. The following visualization works with an outer aspect of the central channel, as it is easier to get initial results. Inner and outer aspects, in this usage, refer more to how deep and subtle our awareness resides. It is also important that the core of the visualization occur physically deep within the body, not around it, or outside of it. The visualization needs to include a connection with the heart, and it should be easy to shift the focus at times to emphasize the navel area.

Begin with a few general warm up exercises of your choosing. Do just enough to energize your sitting and make breathing deep and easy; however, not so much that you are tired. A few simple exercises that help to do this are camel ride, spinal twisting and heart twirl for a few minutes each, perhaps preceded by some martial art kicks and running in place.

If you are already energized you may skip the exercises, or substitute ones of your choice.

Camel Ride

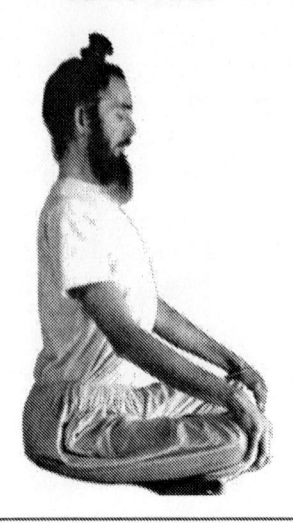

Sitting with the legs crossed, hold onto your ankles and flex the lower spine forward as you inhale, flexing back as you exhale. Develop a fluid motion keeping the head relatively still. As you inhale forward, bring the breath down the front and as you exhale back, bring the breath up the back, particularly through the tailbone. In all these exercises, you breathe through the nose.

When finished, inhale with a straight back and hold the breath for a moderate time while squeezing the anus, contracting the base of the genitals, pulling in the navel and directing energy up the spine.

Spinal Twisting

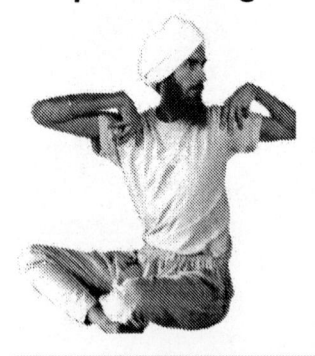

Rest the hands on top of your shoulders with the elbows out to the side: Inhale as you twist to the left, exhale as you twist to the right, revolving around the spine.

Variations include interlocking the hands together facing downwards in front of the chest, interlocking the hands facing downwards above the head, and bringing both arms straight up above the head with palms flat together.

Heart Twirl

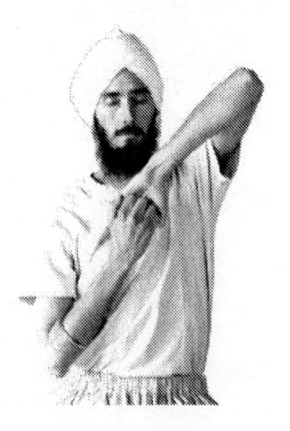

Lock the fingers of each hand together in bear-grip, elbows out to the side. Inhale as you twist the left elbow up and right down, exhale as you twirl the arms the other direction. The hands stay in one place in front of the chest. The arms are like a propeller clearing away obstructions of the heart and breath. As you breathe, build energy in the navel area and let this energy rise to spread out around the chest through the motion of the arms.

Now sit still with a straight spine. Breathe easily with awareness, throughout the body and as you do so feel the three-dimensional space within your body. Sometimes the breath becomes very deep and full. Becoming aware of the soles of the feet, the palms of the hands, and the top of the head helps you to draw in energy and open up. Move the focus around the body. Sometimes you may focus in an area of the spine, or an organ, or the whole body. Breathe like this for five or ten minutes.

As a separate practice, you may breathe like this for as long as desired, even for many hours. This type of breathing, while very simple, is extremely beneficial in developing the Inner Temple. It keeps us very awake, while also internalizing us. Over the years, you will discover many refinements in the playful process of uniting body, breath and mind.

Feel the palms of the hands, soles of the feet and top of the head open more fully. Imagine a sea of energy around you, within you, and available to you. It is like being in a lightning storm on a summer day—there is a charge in the air and you feel alive just being in it. Make sure your navel area is connected.

Lightly connect with your sensual energy. Visualize and feel earth energy, as a fine red mist, spiraling up from beneath you directly into your genitals and through the soles of your feet, up your legs. Feel sexy, without over doing it. The earth energy and your sensual energy are one, spiraling up both around and within you. Bring some of this spiraling mist upward into the heart, as if that is where it is destined to go. The lower back feels connected and strong.

Some of this spiral continues up all the way to the top of your head and even beyond. Develop the sensual, enveloping feeling and you can add your own creative nuances to create that feeling as appropriate. At times, draw your perineum upwards. Remember the dan-tien area several inches below the navel and a few inches inwards, because by empowering this area, you will draw in more energy and transform that energy into nourishment that your body can use.

While doing this, remember to keep breathing and keep a whole-body sense. After a few minutes, simultaneously feel the top of your head become more transparent. From the heavens, bring down a white nectar-light-energy-presence-mist, spiraling through and around your body in the opposite direction of the red mist. Make it sweet—the earth of heaven. As it spirals down, it intertwines with the upward sensual earth energy, principally at the heart, but also with a whole-body feeling. The essences dance in love—a blissful quality that consumes the analytical mind and opens an inner effortless space.

Now, keeping the support of the above, condense this awareness into two tubes of light (one on each side of the spine). Condense the red mist into your right side and give it a feminine quality. Condense the white mist into your left side and give it a masculine quality.[1] Sense this light-nectar intertwining in an upward helix through the center of your body. The helix is about three inches across, but may vary from person to person and at different times. Each cord of the light is about a ¼ inch across, yet there is a larger radiance emanating from each cord. This intertwining has an intense passionate sexual quality to it. You are literally making love within yourself. This helix and the feeling it invokes is the primary focus of this meditation.

After enjoying this sea of bliss for a while, bring your awareness deeper into the center of the heart, right in the middle of that helix. Feel a deep inner space within the heart. Do not focus too much energy, just let it rise from its own side. If in doing this, the sensual sea of bliss disappears, that is ok. Enjoy the quietude and radiant peace within the heart.

The helix that you have awakened is one of the outer aspects of the central channel. Enjoy it, cultivate it, but do not try too hard to keep it always present. Later, as you begin to develop the inner aspect of the central channel, the bliss may initially lessen. This is normal. As you continue, the bliss will eventually come back much greater. While the outer aspect of the central channel can create bliss and remove obstructions of the analytical mind, the inner aspect is liberation itself.

---

[1] You may alternatively condense the feminine red mist into the left side and the masculine white mist onto the right. There are reasons for each approach. However, for this purpose, the intertwining of the two is the most important aspect.

The Inner Temple is the effortless and eternal radiant energy of our existence. The form of energy radiating in the Inner Temple is your true body, interacting with the universe of which you are one. It can turn any mundane experience into divinity. A simple touch, a sight, awareness of a patch of skin, when revealed in this light, is pregnant with ecstasy.

For Those Who Want a Simpler Start

A most important activity is KNOWING YOUR PHYSICAL BODY AS LIGHT. Visualize and feel your heart radiating a bright Golden Light enveloping your body and the space around it with an effortless radiance.

Go within your body, breathe through it and sense or feel a radiance of light within it. To give further definition and opening of the heart, go right into the core of the heart chakra, between the nipples and deep in the chest, a little more towards the back than the front. Radiate from it the sense of purity and bright transparency that comes from relaxing into your own presence. As you improve, outer thoughts will naturally disappear as your consciousness focuses itself through this deeper energy.

Another practice is to feel within the three-dimensional area of your body. Sense your image as radiant light, in exactly the same shape of the body. Be sure to feel the spatial quality of the body, for example, the area inside your chest, within your whole torso, your head, etc. Be aware of yourself as this body of light being normal and aware. Do not project out of yourself, but stay contained and activated. It may help to start by feeling the inside of the body as empty space with a thin, golden skin—later fill the inside with light, and bring more definition to that light until it has all the inner qualities of your body. Starting with a bright red light works well. Feel that red light within your body as you, complete with eyes and self-awareness.

Practice regularly. Some may enjoy it right away, while others may need to work with exercises first, such as the dynamic yoga practices to gain the meditative capacity.

Summary of the First Technique

This is not so much any one specific technique as it is developing a relationship with the body as light. While we could just visualize light, it is more important that this light has a relationship with the body and therefore felt as residing within it. Develop spatial awareness, detail, wholeness, feeling, radiance, purity, connectivity and depth.

You want to become familiar with a feeling of depth and energy in the middle of your body, running up and down it. In the next meditations, we will extend that core up above the head. Because this core is in relationship with your body, you can use the energies of your body as a point of reference—and to stay awake. Using the body as a point of reference is one of the keys of Eternal Yoga practice, whereby we develop symmetrical awareness. This symmetry awareness includes the light above the head in relation to both our body and the central channel as it extends up through the top of our head, as well as of the various presences within our body in relation to our central channel.

In the first technique, we wish to stabilize awareness within the subtle pranas of our central channel. We do so by first purifying and energizing the subtle energies of the body as a whole. As we do this and focus within our central core, we feel the relationship of the body as a whole with our center. This harmony helps us in dynamically remaining centered, i.e., using the vitality of our body as a field of awareness in which we center. While at first we are more aware of the physical pranas, gradually we become stabilized within the subtle pranas that are the central channel, or as termed in the Indian yogas, the spinal marrow and within that the shushumna and within that the vajra channel and within that the chinti channel. That is to say, more and more we feel that we are this subtle energy of our soul emanating out into a physical body, rather than a physical body trying to find something within it.

The above chapter could easily be an introduction to kriya yoga techniques, so I hope that you understand that the first technique of creating the Inner Temple is not one technique in itself, rather a process of increasing vitality, internalization, and identification of oneself more in terms of light and subtle energy.

Always strengthen the foundation of meditating within the body as light. The practices given in the book, *Cultivating a Body of Nectar: Kriya Yoga and Tantric Foundations* are wonderful for this. In addition to the kriyas, expand upon this with explorative meditations of the chakras, channels, energies, and essences, as described in the book. As you discover this for yourself, you can make a play of this with your subtle breath, visualization, and inner sight for hours at a time, experiencing numerous indescribable sensations such as an inner water fountain, vistas of space, and the comforting vitality of energy massaging through your body. Your organs will gain a personality and your body will become a universe with a developing glow deep inside that stays with you through the day, ever-ready for fresh contact and further meditation.

While this can take years to ignite, it will do so if you stay with it. It is a gradual growth, but it is yours.

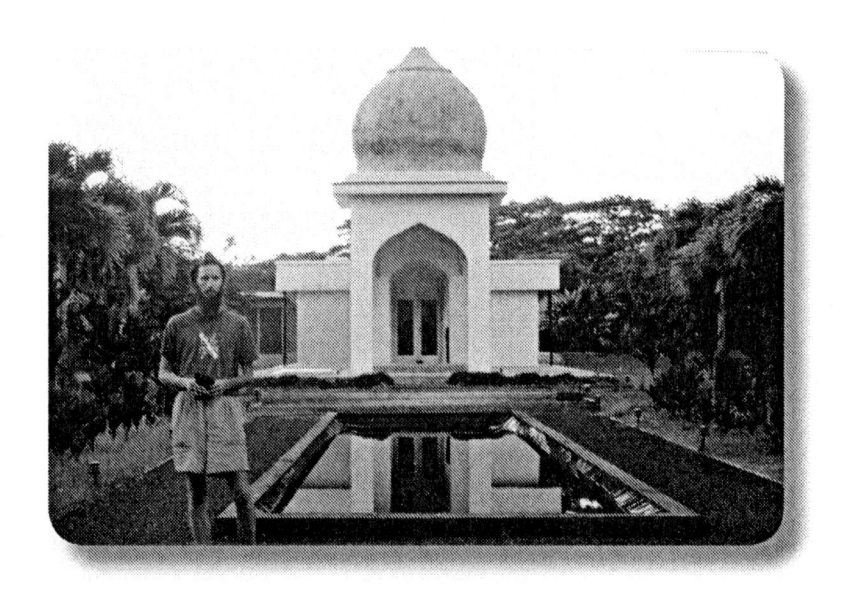

CONNECTING TO YOUR SOURCE OF PRESENCE

This technique is the principle initiatory practice of Eternal Yoga. Mahavatar BabaJi first showed it to me in the 1980's. In summary, his words were, "This is the secret to creating the eternal body." A few years later, I learned that Guy Ballard, who learned it from Saint Germain, taught the essence of this same practice in the 1930's. In my first night in the Himalayas in 1994, Lahiri Mahasaya came in a dream, saying that all his abilities and awareness originated through this meditation, of which he gave me a transmission.

This practice is subtle and if not given importance, most would discard it after an initial curiosity. While it is not necessary to do this meditation for long (ten minutes is enough), do it regularly. In this practice, we will reference a point of consciousness far above the head that becomes the means of sustaining symmetry within the subtle energy body. Awareness of this symmetry is extremely important in overcoming obstructions and self-distortion. In addition, through this point, we open a pathway of initiation from and into higher consciousness. It is a way of keeping the subtle light body aligned with the natural and infinite intelligence of spirit.

As a support for this practice, I recommend starting the session with the meditation previously given on cultivating the Inner Temple. Otherwise, breathe deeply for as long as necessary, directing the presence of each breath into various areas of the body, then center your attention within the heart, feeling an effortless radiance take over.

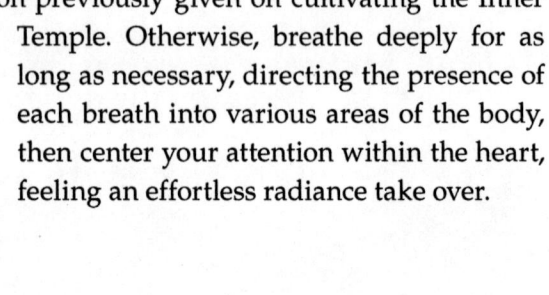

Feel the top of your head open. Feel the area just above your head— then come back down into the body, back and forth a few times so that you feel as if your body has grown in size to include the area above your head. Inwardly look up and sense an uprising of attention, narrowly focused, moving up through the top of your head and continuing for about thirty to fifty feet in a straight line. As you do so, it is very important to remain in your body and connected to it. Do not disassociate from the body. **Do not send up an image of yourself or imagine a beam of light.** *Simply bring forth an intuitive sense, a feeling, of your presence moving up. While doing this, consciously feel that you are reaching up to the pinnacle of your own formless God-essence.*

Pay attention and, at some point in your upward journey, connect to a feeling, a point, a click, something, where you feel your Presence effortlessly radiating down towards your body. It is very subtle, yet noticeable. Remain aware of this invisible light, and particularly the effortless quality in which it emanates from this point down around you.

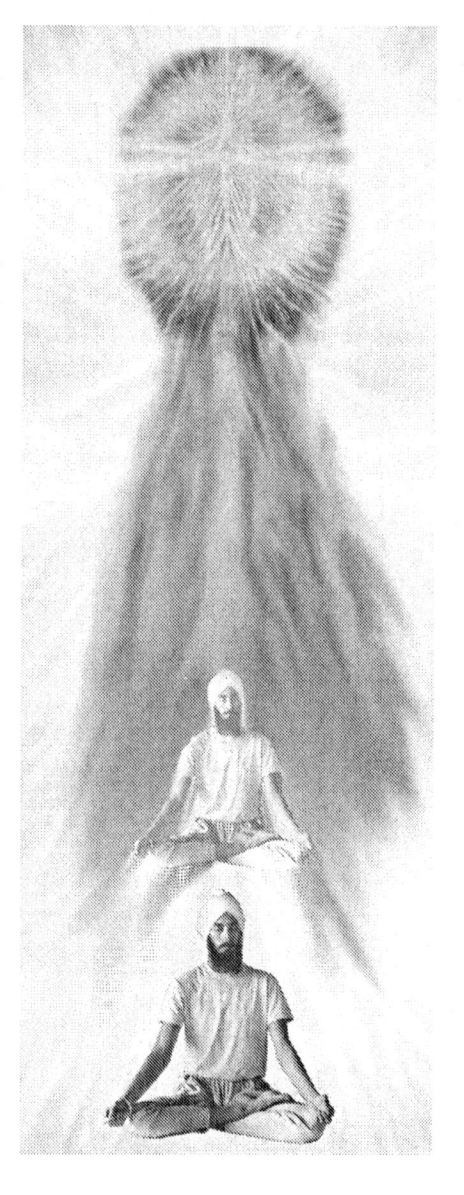

After five or ten minutes, lower your attention to the area above the head. This is where you will develop awareness of your light body, which we will explore in the next meditation on developing the Subtle Body of Light. When finished be sure to bring yourself fully within your physical body.

The point where the energy "clicks" or "bounces back" and returns, is what I call the Tenth Realm[2] or the *Gateway of Purity*. As the gateway into clear light awareness, this point corresponds to what some Tibetan tantras call "The mind of black near-attainment." When entered, it is the same as the clear light entered within the depth of the heart.[3]

Know that you can anchor your highest intentions at this point. It is from this point of reference that you will gain your Victory. Some may spontaneously sense an image originating at that place; for others, it is just a subtle point. With an intention originating from "up there," sense a thick tube of Light moving down, into, and around the body—totally centering it in a feeling of effortlessness, inherent divinity, elevation and higher direction. Be at ease and focused at the same time, going deeper into the absorption of this awareness.

Sense the physical body as Light—bright, strong, translucent and responsive to this effortless light, which is in truth its Source. Feel that this Light from above takes the form of your radiant-physical-body as it descends.

While this point above your head is real, the concept of spatial distance is purely a psychological, yet effective, means of entering it. By going far enough above the head, there is simultaneously a refining of our pranas of awareness. We transcend our personality and grasping nature. In reality, there is nowhere your spirit is not, and traditionally, a practitioner enters into the depths of the heart, often through decades of preliminary practice, to find it as Source.

Often, practitioners fool themselves that they are deep enough in the heart, or the central channel, when in reality they are not. This depth is easier to enter above the head.[4] It will not work to project an image to that point above the head; rather, you must relax in your

---

[2] Some traditions call the crown chakra the tenth gate. Their usage is in reference to the nine orifices or physical openings of the body, with the tenth being the crown of the head. In our usage, we are referencing the major energy gateways of the subtle body, thus the crown chakra would be the seventh and the point in reference here, the tenth.

[3] This (originating deep in the heart) is where I first experienced this state almost a decade earlier. At that time, I was also aware of the various realms above the head coming into an effortless alignment and clarity.

own nature of emptiness, while at the same time not forgetting your physical body. Within this balance lies the truth of existence.

In a number of traditional practices, we try to imagine this subtle experience of emptiness through facsimiles, such as meditating on empty space, or visualizing an empty body, or repeating concepts of emptiness to ourselves—and only very late in the practice is it actually realized. In Eternal Yoga, you literally "touch upon" this experience right from the beginning. This is vital to empowering the understanding of getting there by being there. Without empowerment, it is impossible to practice the inner tantras. The inner tantras are empowered through the feeling that you effortlessly emanate out of emptiness itself into a body of light.

This method allows sincere and advanced practitioners to bypass much of the initial priestly empowerment systems and go direct to further empowerment from the Buddha fields and its inhabitants (the Ascended Masters). This is one of the blessings of Eternal Yoga.

A spontaneously arising awareness can occur from within that point way above the head. These are visions within the clear light of consciousness. However, do not "try" to gain this vision, as it will occur effortlessly.

For this stage of practice, only meditate on this point for short times, and thereafter, allow your meditation to move to other areas such as your body of light directly above the head (which is the subject of the next meditation technique). You do not want to grasp at it, or try to qualify it into anything other than what it is. This is very important. Just keep it simple.

If you imaginatively change it into something that it is not, you will lose the purity of it, and the other practices of going above the head can easily lead you down the path of your own illusions.

Keep in mind, this is a shortcut method to connect with this subtle awareness. For this initial stage of practice, working with this radiant point of awareness is the perfect amount of connection. As

---

[4] The shortcut of going above the head is the way that Saint Germain and Godfrè Ray-King were able to give the essence teaching of non-dualistic awareness to outwardly unprepared Americans in the 1930's. Even so, many distorted the understanding by taking the consciousness of I-AM presented as the inseparable blending of form and emptiness and distorting it to egoic-grasping and projection.

we mature, we will fill in many of the details. Further chapters in this book will address many of the subtleties of this and the other initiatory practices.

Mistakes to Avoid in the Second Technique

The most common mistake in this very important technique is not going far enough above the head. You cannot project an image or experience through this distance to that point. If you do, then you are not going far enough. When you go above the head and stop at about six feet above the head, you can enter a very subtle mental realm, whereby it seems very far up and you can fool yourself that you have found that point, because of the profoundness.

The reason you cannot project an image, is that the image is composed of the pranas of imagination, or the pranas of your personality, which exists within a framework of relative existence. The gateway above your head is a place of the light beyond the light—it is beyond the soul, beyond the personality. You cannot enter it through relative existence. This is the same as saying that you cannot meditate yourself into a Buddha.

For those who are having trouble finding this effortless point of radiance; a guide who truly understands from the level of spirit, and thus can inwardly see your effort, can help guide you by opening up the path and giving you feedback as to what is occurring and where you are at.

If you cannot remain connected to your body doing this practice, then do more yoga exercises, kriyas, and visualizations within the body, such as the initiatory steps of creating the Inner Temple. Your body is a familiar source of energy to stay awake and focused.

Remaining in the body allows you to gauge the distance, and allows the polarity to exist whereby, as we move further up, the subtle pranas of the personality are dropped. By being in the body, you will gradually feel the effortless radiance from deep in the heart. In the tantras, you will enter this same awareness, in totality, directly within the heart itself.

Without a purity of intention in the heart, you will not find this gateway. The ego wants more importance than it truly has, and the humility of such a seemingly inconsequential and non-phenomenal point having more importance is not easy for some. While initiating people in this practice, I am inwardly aware of their results. If there is something about yourself that you do not want to see, it will be difficult to find the point. You are opening yourself to the raw purity of truth, and if we have very deep investments in keeping our illusions intact, then we create a subtle resistance to this effect.

Another common mistake is doubt, "I think I experienced it, but I am not sure." Do not make it more, do not make it less; just connect, and leave your thoughts out of the process. There is a way of overcoming this doubt, in that while it seems like nothing has happened, the memory of that connection and the effortless raining back of subtle awareness has a way of staying with you whereas an imaginary event would have vanished quickly.

This meditation opens a path for certain additional transmissions that cannot easily occur otherwise. Without maintaining the purity of that point, the subtle ego in its desires can and often does override the wisdom of spirit.

Closing Remarks on the Second Technique

Of course, Spirit is everywhere and everything. What we are awakening to, we are already. It is easy to use the word spirit, in a spirited conversation. Yet when it comes down to the practicality of working with your spirit in the context of liberation—it can be a slippery subject. There is often confusion as to what spirit is. For some people it is anything other than the physical; some confuse spirit and soul; for some people, it is a voice in their head, "Spirit told me so," or a vague feeling, or moments of feeling peaceful. To be effective, we must truly know what spirit is, beyond any doubt. We need to find our spirit, the dharmakaya, in a pure, direct manner, and in the continuum of our existence. When we know spirit, the underlying nature of our existence, we rest in it.

To know ourselves as spirit, we need to get out of our own way. The problem is, most people do not know how to get out of their own way. Even if we want to, it is always me thinking, me not thinking, me doing something or me not doing something. Always the me trying to escape does no good; it is still within a relativistic framework. Going to sleep is simply going to sleep—we wake up in the same condition. Even when we do experience the perfection of spirit, we do not know how to remain in it, or how to bring it back—we grasp after it and thus only make ourselves unaware of it again. We can forget about it for many lifetimes—caught in the limits of our personality is like living for a million years and nothing advances. Spirituality remains a religion, an ideal, an idea, a morality, or perhaps a good phase of experiencing the heart. In love, we enjoy life, and at least we temporarily heal the hurts of our separation. Yet most of us do not, or cannot, rest in it long and deep enough. We end up qualifying it, again, in the context of the prison of ourselves.

This meditation opens the doors of spiritual realization, by which further successes can occur. Of the many and infinite ways we become aware of spirit in relation to our physicality, Eternal Yoga is one of the most effective and, for the average person, perhaps one of the quickest ways. It is practical and a very conscious means of entering into the enlightened view.

The nature of non-dual transmissions occurs within the oneness, from teacher to student, primarily in two ways. The most direct way is a total dissolving of all the pranas into the central channel at the heart. The transmission of the movement of pranas may start years in advance. There is no mistake as to what is happening—it is a cosmic and total event. There are very few who have the capacity for this level of transmission and practice; however, the Eternal Yoga practices are a step towards this capacity.

A more common level of transmission, available to a larger number of practitioners, occurs in a subtle context, along with the physical or telepathic communication as to the importance of what is occurring, amidst the backdrop of many other subtleties. Initiation of a student into Eternal Yoga practice would be within this context.

In truth, many have had enlightened moments. Yet, because of the simplicity of the moment, few know the true value of these experiences, or how to cultivate them. The Eternal Yoga practices aim to bring forth the simplicity of this experience, nothing mind-blowing, and teach us to value it, and thus slowly cultivate ourselves into a continuance.

As a perspective of consciously applying ourselves to awaken, versus simply waiting for it, a Master, physical or subtle, may give a momentary transmission to millions of people in the course of a lifetime—such as clearly seeing the aliveness and divinity of this point radiating within each person in a crowd simultaneously. To give you an idea of the rarity of the success of this type of transmission, perhaps one or two within that lifetime will gain and maintain significant consciousness of it.

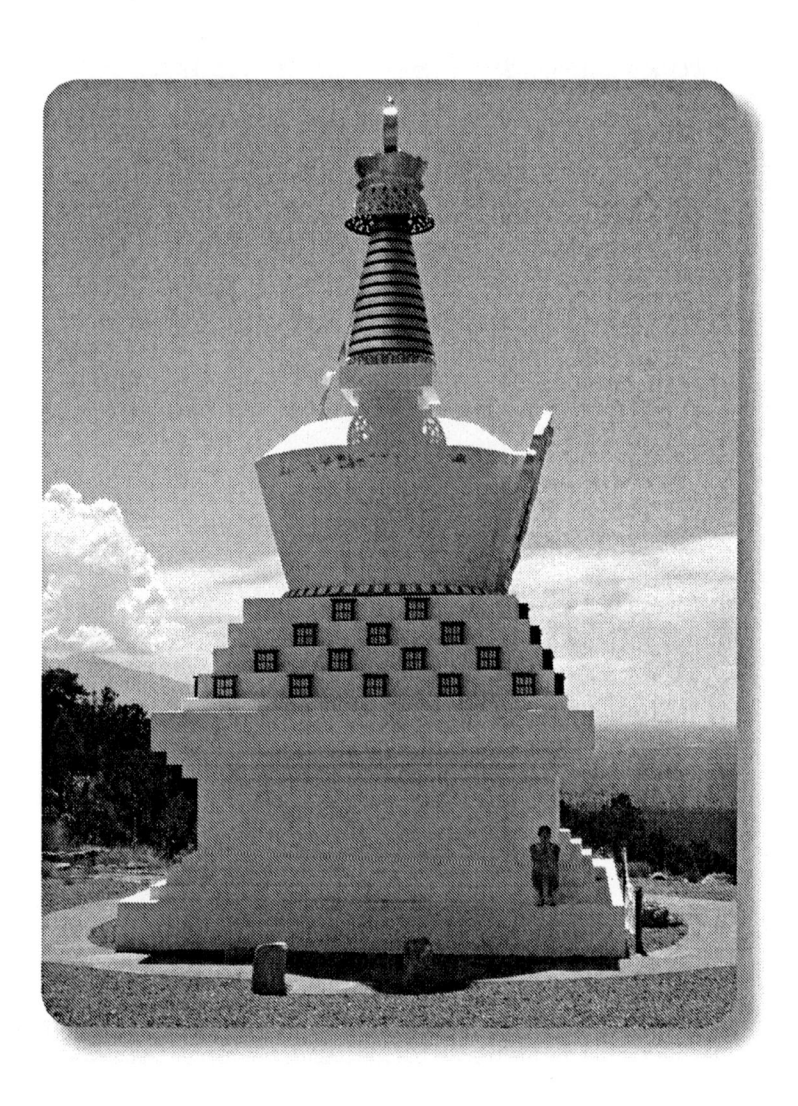

THE SUBTLE BODY OF LIGHT

We form our subtle body of light out of the effortless pranas of spirit. In the Eternal Yoga practices, we will do this above our head. Within the Eternal Yoga practices, the majority of our meditative time is this practice. Later in the tantric practices, we will experience it within the central channel, and thus directly underlying everything in the physical as well.

In Buddhist terminology, this subtle body of light is the sambhogakaya body (enjoyment or bliss body), the body of a Buddha, or the illusory body. In the west, we call it our soul.

We all live in a world made out of many types and levels of energy. For example, we have various energies that emanate from our thoughts, emotions, and tissues that form a temporary energy body. This is not what we mean by the subtle body of light. The true subtle body of light is composed of pranas that emanate out of pure consciousness, out of empty space. They are not from what we eat, or how we feel after work, or projections of our mind from this kind of consciousness. Our subtle body of light, while capable of constant change, exists beyond conventional understandings of birth and death, and when truly understood, becomes an eternal body.

Always begin your practice by first touching in with the point way, way above the head as previously described. Now focus a few inches above your head. Imagine, feel, sense, visualize a focus of light there. In the beginning, this is enough. Be sure to remain connected within your body while doing this, and when you finish drop your energy fully down into the body. The effect is to feel as if you have grown in height to include a few inches above your head. This area just above the head I call the realm of *creative harmonization*. The eighth center[5] creates, in seed form, all of the primary energy patterns of the body—for example: the spinal current, the frontal channel, the central channel, and the primary chakras.

The next area to explore is from three to six feet above the head. This area I call *seeing by becoming*. The ninth realm is of the higher mental body. Here you can easily connect to collective currents. The subtlety of your mind can project, become, and bless. It is from here that a yogi can be in many places at once (in subtle awareness). One way to begin to awaken awareness of this realm is to visualize a collection of light and within it an eye of seeing. Make this small, say from an inch to four or five inches in total.

In awakening within these centers, there is a lot of play involved. We begin by using already familiar ways of staying awake, such as how we see light, familiar images, feelings, etc., and project these above. For example, we might visualize riding a horse, but do so above our head, we may visualize ourselves sitting in meditation above our head, or we may visualize our image of a particular guide above our head.

Wherever there is prana, there is a support for consciousness. Thus, we use this to stay awake. Of course, this projection is not the true light of these realms, but it is a way to begin to hold a focus in the ballpark. Because we are moving above our head, there is automatically a mechanism of refinement in effect. Eventually, we start to transfer awareness into the pranas that originate from within these realms themselves. As we do that, we gain a true awareness.

As we awaken above the head, we are opening Pandora's Box. Within our soul is a collection of all our experiences, particularly our root attitudes and beliefs we have developed within our soul through our experiences and reflection. The light of our soul is either the direct cause of that which binds us in endless existence, or that which brings us to the gates of liberation. Through cultivating willingness to see and the ability of penetration, we can see in hours or days that which can otherwise take lifetimes to unveil. Until a person enters

---

[5] In describing the realms above the head, I often use the words: realm, chakra, and center, seemingly interchangeably. A chakra or center is a focus within a realm. While a center tends to denote a focus solely within that realm, a chakra is also the outpouring of the energies into other realms, i.e., like a bridge or meeting place. Think of how the sun radiates the intense reality of its existence, through its rays, into many different worlds that are of a different nature. To center within the sun, is to be in the reality of the sun. Thus, we most easily enter into these rarified realms (from our denser existence) through a point of focus.

This terminology works perfectly well in the eighth and ninth centers, as this helps us to develop a continuum of this consciousness into the physical. For the eleventh and twelfth realms, the concept of a fixed center, or a chakra, disappears; thus, if I use the term, center or chakra, in this context, it is simply for comfort in trying to describe the indescribable.

this level of soul awareness, there is no chance of liberation within a relatively short time, such as within one lifetime.

Our ability to succeed depends on the purity of the anchor developed through the second technique. It also depends on the infallible connection we create to the ascended body. Some Buddhist traditions further classify our awareness through the soul body as being either an impure or a pure illusory awareness. The impure illusory awareness is activity through this body of light while remaining ignorant that it is an emanation from our spirit. It is like basking in the warmth of the sun, ignorant that the light and heat has originated from the sun. We claim it as our own and look upon it as a subtle personality complete in itself, ignorant of the Body of the One and the true nature of our spirit. In contrast, the pure illusory body is a body of light that is aware of its source in the effortless and ever-flowing nature of spirit. The pure illusory body is the body of a Buddha. Always infinitely tuned to the greater spirit—we directly express ever-expanding perfection in full clarity.

In developing our body of light, we have so far only uncovered the tip of the iceberg. Almost the entire remainder of this book, directly or indirectly, addresses further development of this awareness, along with pitfalls to watch for and ways of integration. There is more than could fit in a book, and there are aspects that are highly personal. It is important, at various times, that you receive direct, competent guidance for this journey.

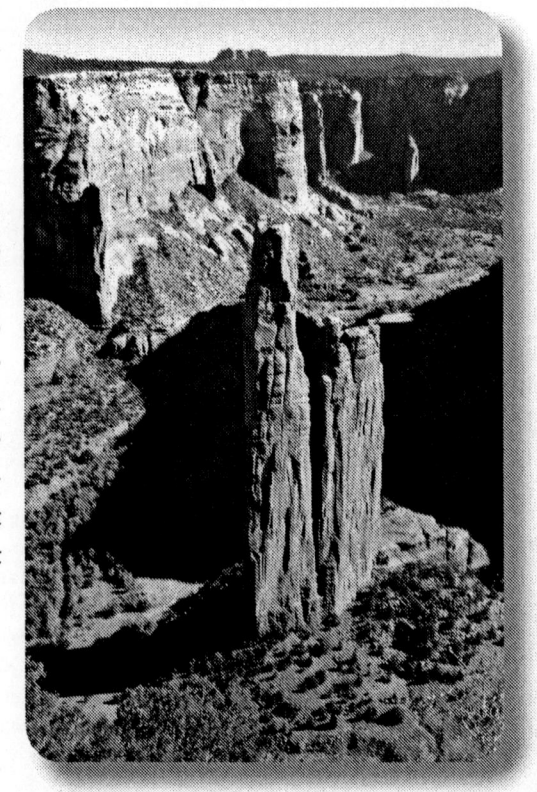

HEALING INTO PERFECTION

I AM, this day and every day, EVER-EXPANDING PERFECTION

Make this your first thought upon awakening, while keeping the feeling of it in the heart. An advanced practitioner may simply remain with the non-verbal radiation of their Inner Temple.

This affirmation keeps the energy of your spirit connected to your every-day reality. It helps in eliminating doubt and strengthens awareness of the radiant-mind. Take care that you feel this affirmation emanating from beyond your ego-nature, otherwise, it will simply increase arrogance.

This affirmation facilitates a vision of the enlightened fabric of ascended consciousness underlying everything. It opens your heart and is very healing. It releases the energy of judgment that may be holding you back. It is humbling. When conjoined with penetration, it helps us to rest in what flows from the highest levels of our being. As a mantra of awareness, it checks the nature of the un-enlightened personality to re-qualify[6] this perfection into something else. This affirmation says that the universe is a dynamic, constantly growing, constantly evolving, interdependent activity. It is very personal and intimate. This transparency is vital for the play of the inner tantras.

At times, I find myself singing this mantra, and experiencing a beatific vision in which everything is divine; outwardly, bad or good, dirty or clean, love or hate, it all has something within it that sings of the underlying fabric of divinity.

---

[6] The highest levels of our being are always qualifying the original light of spirit into something. Without this, we do not exist. It is impossible to separate the two, the light of spirit and its original qualities. This is not a vague light, rather: blissful, infinitely exact, and containing all possibilities from beginningless time, of which there is a predominant awareness of Perfection. As this light, so to speak, filters down into the fabric of our forgetful creation, we tend to "re-qualify" this light into something more suitable for the needs of our immediate personality, i.e., one of the lesser possibilities of the infinite landscapes existing in this light.

Part of the skillful activities of a spiritual adept, is helping people not to, or in certain instances, not to allow, the requalification of the higher realities of this light. As a simple example of the personality re-qualifying what they know to be true; consider building a house in a place where you know nothing should be built, yet you want a house there anyway.

The tremendous vista of the soul is something that unfolds over time. This requires the prerequisite understanding that everything occurring in your life, including difficulties, is there for a reason. There are no accidents. This puts you in the place to see, to learn, and to move forward in the Ever-Expanding Perfection.

"This day and everyday," is the eternal nature of your spirit beyond the limits of external time. Watch yourself that you do not try to grasp at the affirmation. The "I," your identity, must flow into, from, and through the rest of the affirmation; otherwise, it is just projecting your limited personality. You want it to be like saying, "God is, this day and everyday, the Ever-Expanding Perfection." If in this context you then boast, "I Am God," that is a stupid and ego-centered attitude. If you say, God is not me, but out there, this is also ignorance. Rather, you have to surrender into it. There is sacredness in it. To achieve this you have to dissolve past your immediate personality and deepen into the truth and purity of effortlessly radiance. In all honesty, it is you as spirit, not you as limited personality, which can truly make this affirmation. That is what you want to connect with and affirm through this attunement.

While the results of this affirmation should include a greater harmony and lightness, be careful not to become blind to your problems or the world's troubles at large. At the same time, do not let problems make you blind to the underlying reality of spirit, for this is simply strengthening the trap of our un-enlightened view. A mature perspective is feeling and knowing at all times the underlying spirit, light, and perfection within every moment, and thus being in touch with a divine view, and a creative force in us that evolves the world and us simultaneously. This affirmation helps us to remember that space which we experience in our enlightened moments.

We are not becoming passive, rather simultaneously active and in great peace. For example, real compassion may include the use of skillful means that outwardly can appear manipulative or destructive. What about killing a man who is trying to kill a hundred with a machine gun, or stopping a child against their adamant wishes who is about to step into traffic, or the wisdom of a person smoking who is just trying to keep their head above water? Are not all of these actions also, in a relativistic sense, perfection? Moreover, what about all the obviously unfair and downright mean things that happen in the world?[7] Are we to become blind and uncaring?

This affirmation is not about becoming unconscious, but about becoming a directness of the ever-expanding nature of spirit into creation, i.e., the "I am" of the affirmation. We are becoming a positive, life-giving energy that has direct insight and wisdom at its service, able to transform the world into a better place, starting with ourselves. Thus, in the process of difficulties, we do not lose the vision of overcoming ordinary appearances. *This is the primary gift of this affirmation, putting into practice overcoming ordinary appearances.*[8] Not just as a passive meditation, but also as an active reality. Without this, ascension is just a word and divinity just an emotional belief.

I AM THE EVER-EXPANDING PERFECTION

---

[7] In addition, what about unfairness to us? There are times on the spiritual path where either for our purification, or to help us be aware of certain things, or in the process of creating change, or helping others of whom we are not separate, or forcing us to ground deeper, unfairness is heaped upon us in unusually large doses. In the right framework, all this can be seen as a learning, and ultimately experienced, as a blessing. If we try to fit the spiritual path into the rules of the unenlightened-mind, we are not in the necessary depth to be on this path.

[8] The result of overcoming ordinary appearances, of absolute solidity, is the enlightened view.

Reality from the Higher Realms

The book, *Cultivating a Body of Nectar*, presents wisdom for exploring our subtle anatomy within the body (see Chapter five, Chakras, Channels, Energy and Essences). In Eternal Yoga, we introduce ourselves to the realms above the head.

I spontaneously began this exploration in 1984 and found five distinct realms of consciousness above the head. At the time of discovery (remembering), I had no external reference for what I was experiencing, so I coined the terminology used here.

In understanding how all this integrated as a continuum into our physical existence, I experienced twelve primary realms, orchestrated within four octaves, with three aspects within each octave. From the bottom up, the first aspect of each octave is the gateway, principally a feeling or emotional quality. The second aspect is principally etheric, containing energetic patterns and images of form, like a template made out of energy. The third aspect is principally mental or spacious in nature.

The accompanying diagram displays this relationship. The focus of each realm into our being results in a chakra. For example, within the second octave, the *Integration of Form*, the Heart chakra forms as the gateway, the Throat chakra expresses the template, and the Third Eye chakra is the mental aspect.

I sometimes use words like "the natural seat" or "the natural tendency," when referring to a chakra or octave as they are not limited to their dominant theme. For example, we can experience all the realms within the Heart chakra. Because of this nature of Oneness, there are many different ways we can chart the relationship of its various, ever-changing components.

Often, a particular way of describing the relationship of various chakras and energies is only useful within the intended context of its use. Thus, the descriptions given in this chapter are most pertinent to the understanding of Eternal Yoga and Tantric practice, in particular to help the integration of our very subtle awareness into the energy fabric of our body. It is like a map of the world: good for getting a perspective, and vital for understanding which direction to go when visiting another country. This map is of little use when all we want is to visit our neighbor in the next town over.

Reality from the Higher Realms 63

Twelve Seats of Consciousness

Singularity of
SPIRIT

Mental
Emotional! *Etheric*

12. Creation of Possibility

11. Divine Personification.

12. Gateway of Purity

9. Seeing by Being

8. Creative Harmonization

7. Gateway of Oneness

6. Understanding within Separation

5. Mastery of Form

4. Gateway of Love

3. Individual Will

2. Creative Impulse

1. Strength

Patterning of Form

Beyond the Light

Orientation of Form

The Soul

Integration of Form

Emotional Seat

Stabilization of Form

Physical Anchor

While, it is more accurate to start from the top of the chart down, for purposes of already existing familiarity, I will start from the bottom up.

The lowest octave is the *Stabilization of Form*, which is the natural seat of the physical, containing the navel, sexual, and root chakras. The next octave up is the *Integration of Form* containing the heart, throat and third eye chakras. These two octaves contain the abodes of consciousness and sources of energy relevant for the lives of most people and our foundational practices. The nature of these chakras and how to meditate within them is explored in depth through the book, *Cultivating a Body of Nectar: Kriya Yoga and Tantric Foundations*.

The Octave of Orientation of Form

The first octave above the head is the *Orientation of Form*. This octave is the natural residence for the images of our existence, as they exist in light, independent of the need of a physical body or external nourishment. This living light is our soul. These are the realms of what the Buddhists call the Sambhogakaya Body, or the Enjoyment/Bliss Body.

This is the octave that you will spend the vast majority of your time with in the Eternal Yoga practices. In tantric practice, you will feel this same awareness originating in the body. This is one of the reasons that Eternal Yoga practices makes possible tantric practice—for without experiencing the refinement and nature of this energy, you will not bring forth or be able to connect with the proper core in which to practice.

Guidance in working within this octave is one of the primary reasons for having a competent teacher. It is important that you understand the difference between these realms and spirit. It is so very important that you maintain your connection to the purity of source, your spirit. A teacher can help guide and protect you during this time, provided you listen, while you are learning to understand the difference between these endless realms of light and the purity and ultimate source of spirit itself. It is very subtle, and the difference between true liberation and false liberation.

The Gateway of Oneness

From a bodily perspective, our entrance into this awareness is the crown chakra at the top of our head. Focusing our attention at the crown chakra can be a very expanding experience. I sometimes call this chakra, the *Gateway of Oneness*.

There are a few aspects of the crown chakra to be aware of. The first is the pineal gland in the center of the head. This gland receives light and energy from the crown chakra and focuses it into an alignment in our body. So-called mind-expanding drugs, in general, cause the pineal gland to become misaligned. Marijuana is particularly damaging in this effect. It is difficult, if not impossible, to progress in the Eternal Yoga practices and a number of the kriyas if a significant drug residue is still in your system.

There are a number of kriyas and practices to help realign the pineal gland, such as the Kriya of Five Sounds.[1] Fruits, such as figs and bananas help in this regard as well. Bananas also help to remove residues that are stuck in the lower back of the head. Developing more precision in your life, taking pride in what you do, keeping your energy balanced and connected to the earth, remaining in integrity, earning your keep, having an open mind—all of these help keep your pineal gland healthy.

As we open up the top of our head, we are opening into a huge field of energy. A healthy pineal gland absorbs this energy from above the head as nourishment for the body. It not only absorbs the energy, but enables us to direct this nourishment to other parts of the body as well. Opening up the top of the head gives us easier access to the Masters and our Higher Self; however, we also have easier access to a Pandora's Box of beings, thoughts and energies. The pineal gland helps us to maintain a proper direction and alignment. Without this, we do not have the necessary discrimination, nor are we able to point our boat in the right direction. Thus, we easily become misled.

The ability to develop a practical continuum between the higher realms and our physical body is one of the greatest gifts of having

---

[1] The Kriya of Five Sounds is included in the book, *Cultivating a Body of Nectar: Kriya Yoga and Tantric Foundations* (see Appendix).

a body. Through this continuum, we have a much greater chance of developing the depth of definition needed to become fully awake. We also have a much greater chance to see and change our blind spots. Without the stable orientation of a physical body, our thoughts and reactions can create a whirlwind effect. The body is like a womb in which to birth our consciousness in a stable manner. It is important to realize just how precious a body is for this purpose.

To open the heavenly aspect of the crown chakra, first sit for a while aligning the chakras within your body. Feel an exactness of the navel energy, the opening of the heart, and the mystical depth of the throat. Sense that the top of your head, the palms of your hands, and the soles of your feet are opening, so that through them you can breathe cosmic energy that surrounds you. Then feel the center of your head, between your ears, for a few minutes. This further activates your pineal gland. Now firmly press the tongue up to the back of your palette, towards the throat. Turn your eyes up and feel that you are looking up through the top of your head. After you have the feeling, you can relax the eyes and maintain the feeling itself. Do all of this gently, so that you remain soft. Let your mind become absorbed in the energy and sensation itself, i.e., transcend the chit-chat personality. Rest in this. You may have a sense of transcending the body altogether, or losing awareness of it. This is ok for this exercise.

When you finish, be sure to stretch you hands up, move the body a bit. Bring yourself back down into your navel area, by focusing there. It is a good idea to massage your scalp and face for a minute or so, then stroke the energy down you frontal line a few times. Do not rush off to do some activity, rather, remain silent for at least ten minutes and go for a walk, stretch the body, or take a short nap. Give time to integrate.

You may decide do skip the Eternal Yoga initiatory techniques given in the previous chapter for a few weeks, and simply focus on opening your crown chakra. This will then make it easier to do the other practices.

The Chakra of Creative Harmonization

Going a few inches to about three feet above the head is the realm of *Creative Harmonization*. Of course, you could project an image of yourself above the head, yet this does not necessarily mean you are entering this realm. It could simply be a wandering of your imagination. You need to cultivate *the sense of centering in that place* a few inches above your head, while simultaneously keeping a connection in your body. You could enter this realm above the head and from it project an image of yourself the size of a house. The distances above the head have rhyme and reason only in relation to particulars of relationship with your physical energy body and its central energy channel.

There are several ways of centering yourself in this area above the head. Most of the time, go the route of the Eternal Yoga initiatory techniques, that is: prepare the body, go up to the point way above the head, then drop down to the area just above the head. Sometimes, just simply open up the crown and expand up a few inches, skipping the part of first going way up.

As you are able to feel yourself simultaneously centered above the head, and also in the body, the heart for example, then you will have relaxed enough to experience the subtlety of this realm. Play with it. If you have an area of the physical body that is not well, from above the head, see and feel it as perfect, then cultivate that image and feeling into the same place in the body. You want to feel that the image above your head and the location in your body is, in essence, the same location.

This is a tremendously important chakra for regeneration of the body. From here, you can learn to precipitate indescribable nectars down into the body. Sometimes, you can experience instantaneous healings.

To work with nectar, you need to bring forth a tangible quality to light. A good training for this is to first develop this ability at the third eye. Practice gathering enough attention at the third eye area to gather prana into that area. You will feel the sensation of it. Now soften and sweeten the prana, so that it does not create any dullness, headiness, or pain from longer periods of focus. The ability to focus at the third eye in a soft manner occurs over repeated practice sessions.

Practice inhaling and exhaling energy and light through the third eye into the body. Allow this to occur in a gentle way. Now shift the emphasis to inhaling light in through the third eye and gathering it there as you exhale. At the same time, also make sure to breathe down into the body, so that energy is not stuck in the upper chest. As you gather light essence at the third eye, do so about a half-inch under the skin. Feel a soft, white liquid light gather. Sometimes, sense that white liquid light is rolling up the nose as you inhale into the third eye.

Gently let this liquid, as it builds, move into the bones of the forehead and around the eyes. This feels good. In the primary focus of the third eye, allow the energy of this liquid light to support an image, such as a miniature you. Feel very alive and happy in this miniature you. You are learning how to qualify light into a tangible experience.

As you gather this liquid light, you may direct some of it down into the body. You can nourish any organ, such as your kidneys with it. As you do so, you will also gain greater harmony and strength in the body. When you direct the energy down to an area of the body, also spend some time just focusing in that area on its own. For example, if you are nourishing your tailbone area, then also practice breathing energy up from the earth into your tailbone, and centering there a bit. You want all sides of the relationship to feel their part.

The same way you experience light becoming tangible at the third eye, you can also do in the eighth chakra above the head. There is a natural resonance of this chakra with the throat and sexual centers. You can use any color of light, however, one of the gifts of opening into this realm is learning how to use the Silver Ray. The Silver Ray is like cosmic semen in its power and it is very transcendental. You have to be careful to keep this energy deeply centered. Otherwise, it can create headaches and disturbances in the body, as it is too high of a voltage for the body to handle. This ray can also make you feel like throwing all boundaries to the winds, including marriages, commitments, and social constraints—be careful.

The eighth center has within it, in seed form, all the primary flows of energy present within the physical body. The primary conduit for this is the central channel. Out of the central channel originates the spinal and frontal flows and other flows of energy in the body. Within these flows are specific focal points that become the primary chakras. Because it is a living template for the body, we can rejuvenate and heal the body through strengthening this template and its relationship with our body.

There is a scriptural saying that we carry the karmas of seven generations within our tissues. Our life experiences changes the cellular templates of the body, the DNA. Thus, we inherit, through our DNA, the life experiences of our ancestors. It is not that the genetic strands of DNA are stored in the eighth center; rather, the experience that causes them to be shaped or patterned in a particular way is stored.

Through focusing within the eighth center, we can start to activate some of these experiences. This brings them into our life, which gives us the opportunity to heal those experiences that need healing. In reawakening into the joy of light and the sense of perfection from this center, we can begin to reawaken the energy of this template.

We can start to break the patterns that keep us stuck. If we always get in the same fight, again and again, or do the same stupid things repeatedly, it is as if we are stuck on a track. Of course, there are all sorts of emotional hooks and paybacks for doing this, yet this knowledge does not always help us. Often we need to address a deeper root, which no amount of psychological feedback will help with. Touching in with the eighth centers gets us out of our immediate personality enough to step out of the rut. We can bring forth the authority within us, the deeper permission, to create change. It is empowering ourselves.

From the eighth center, you start to develop the definition of your light body. At first you are projecting and visualizing, a kind of imagination, however, after a period, you will awaken in a tangible presence of effortless light from within the pranas of the buddhic realms. It is no longer an imagination. In this way, you will truly know that you are beyond death. Developing definition within these realms is the subject of next chapter, *Developing the Body of Light*.

The Realm of Seeing by Becoming

From three to six feet above the head is a mental realm, *Seeing by Becoming*. The primary way of seeing in this realm is not with light, but with direct awareness itself. For example, you could describe the texture and color of a suit a friend is wearing and the location of the table near him, without actually seeing any of it. This is a much richer way of seeing, as it is not limited to three dimensions. When you learn to see in this way, you break free of conventional limitations. For example, you can be in multiple places at once. You can simultaneously be aware of many levels of activity at once and know things that are unexplainable through any external vision.

This realm is extremely transcendent of the body. Once awakened to it, this level of transcendence actually makes it easy to work simultaneously in this realm, as you go about your daily business in the physical. Part of awakening to these realms is the willingness to see and know.

It is in this realm that the infinitely responsive mind often makes a connection first into something of relevance for the individual. This is a supreme realm of transmission. For example, I have been aware of thousands of beings, each as an individual, at once. Another time, I saw 12,000 dragons simultaneously, inseparable from the Mandala of my being, and where they were within the planet. I have many times placed the scintillating, golden light of awakening into various hearts, all in perfection. Countless thousands of conversations have occurred with various Masters within the Body of the One. I have been in the secrets of temples beyond outer concept, and the magic done within them. I have experienced stars as sensual consorts and bliss beyond the capacity of a physical body to fathom. You can weave through and create the fabric of time. Even with all this and many more countless experiences, I can say that it is not the phenomenal experiences that I remember, rather the simple beingness of it. If you try to go after the phenomena too much, you will miss this.

If nothing else, remember the simplicity and forget about trying to experience anything in particular. Think of the simplicity of space, of just being, and of love—no reason is necessary.

In these realms, there is an effortless blending with each other. We can become the form of an Ascended Master, and they of us. Without connection, nothing happens at all. You will understand what a Mandala of Enlightened Beings is.

Unfortunately, those who have momentary experiences of these realms overshadowing their normal awareness often cannot understand what is occurring. For example, in feeling oneself as Jesus, the person then goes about and tells everyone they are Jesus.

These realms are not the same experiences of the more common subtle realms, for example, lucid dreaming, LSD trips, mushroom experiences, etc. However, if you know how, you can lift yourself from those realms into these.

It is in the eighth and ninth realms whereby we either bind ourselves or bring forth the grace of liberation. The karmas are extremely subtle, yet the effects far reaching. While this experience is transcendent of the physical, it is important that you are able to develop a continuum into the physical. This continuum is more than just having two separate experiences, one in the ninth realm and one in the physical, which happen to be occurring at the same time. You have to feel the connection between them.

There is simply not enough force of polarity in these subtle realms to draw our attention to mistaken views. In fact, even the concept of a mistaken view does not exist. However, by connecting this subtle realm into a continuum with the physical, there is a chance for the polarities to play out in our life. This makes it easier to see what we want to change about ourselves.

By developing this continuum, we not only develop a definition of our light body that is beyond the death of our physical body, but we also have practice in connecting this to the physical, and can thus better maintain a continuum of awareness in the physical, between one lifetime and the next.

By bringing forth this continuum, we further overcome a dualism that makes it easier to go on to our next step. Without this, we are blind that there is even anything more. Many advanced practitioners consider their experience in this realm the ultimate.

These are the realms of the Gods, which is another experience in cyclic existence, which often lasts for many eons. Do not think of the Gods as gross beings, they are infinitely more refined than that. Often the biggest cause of becoming trapped in these realms is the desire body getting out of control. Through enough meditative effort, skillful application, and merit, anyone can bring themselves forth into these realms. However, to go beyond this, transcends the individual, thus you cannot reach this consciousness through an individual effort. You have to release the grasping and conceptualizing nature.

These realms are also the active realms of the Ascended Masters and Buddhas. It is all the same light, yet with differences in subtle degrees of realization, and thus the ability to respond and work within the perfection.

Patterning of Form Octave

A common description in the scriptures is that the pranas of the eight and ninth realms are like rays of sunlight emanating from your spirit, the sun, the dharmakaya. When you fully enter into the sambhogakaya experience, the body of bliss, it can seem like the ultimate. Yet, there is still a subtle level of separation, a dualism. You can try to meditate yourself beyond it, but no matter how long or how intense you try to do so, it just is, or so it appears.

The next octave above the head is the *Patterning of Form*. It is the home of the Body of the One. It is the light-beyond-light, form-beyond-form. The Buddhists call it Dharmakaya. It is not something that you can enter through technique or ambition, rather something that you already are and awaken into, as you are ready. Those who are awake within the Body of the One give the transmission of it. The truths here are beyond the ability of those in limited consciousness to re-qualify into something else, and it is from here that the Ascended Masters hold the templates of their plans upon the earth.

The Gateway of Purity

The gateway to this octave is the tenth realm, the *Gateway of Purity*. This is the point of spirit that you reference in "the connecting to source" initiatory practice of Eternal Yoga. While we use the omniscient radiance of the tenth realm as "a point" of reference, actually entering through it is another matter altogether. This is what the Buddhists call, "Passing through the black light of near attainment," and on the other side is the clear light of consciousness.

Some Tibetan dharma books erroneously state that it is impossible not to lose consciousness as your move through this realm to the other side, or else it is ideal that one does so (go unconscious) to truly have the experience of the other side. The subtle ignorance of a linear mind creates the experience in this way. The reason that most practitioners go unconscious is that the relative pranas of conventional consciousness, even those in the sambhogakaya realm, cannot pass through this barrier. If you are aware of primal space as the mind itself, prior to its qualifications, then you can go through this apparent barrier with non-dual awareness—as you are already there. This is my own experience. Whether you pass through consciously or not, doing so in totality is unmistakable. Nothing compares to it. The illusion of you, as a distinct atom of the universe, an indivisible personality—disappears; you see the illusion as it is. Once you experience the light beyond the light, you are always there, deep within the heart.

I call the tenth realm the *Gateway of Purity*, as once entered, you are in a state beyond separation. If within this realm you judge what an apparent-another is doing, a Hitler for example, you will become it. There must be enough definition to be awake and be who you are in the universe, while at the same time seeing the perfection of every other form. Only those who live in the purity of spirit can be in this way. Words themselves cannot communicate the fullness, but it is a good start.

The Eleventh and Twelfth Realms

The eleventh realm, I call the realm of *Divine Personification*. It is the form beyond form. The twelfth realm is the *Creation of Time and Space* from its most primal level. Space, in this instance, is the mind itself, and time is feeling itself.

Whenever the Masters bring a soul under the Ascended Body, that person is receiving initiation from these levels, although very, very, few are aware of it in this way. Initiation is an introduction. From this level, you are also subtlely being anchored into a place of no return. You are on your way home. Adeptship is the competent ability to work within this awareness. All of the Ascended Masters are twelfth-level adepts. There are currently only eight beings in physical-human incarnation on the planet, not yet fully ascended "into" the physical, who are twelfth-level adepts.

Adepts at this level, while they can appear as simple people, in the big picture, have been and are involved with the formation of the planet itself. For example, Tara created areas of the Hawaiian Islands, Shiva created the Himalayas, etc.

From this level of consciousness, you are eternally awake. There is nothing to prove, nowhere to go. While existing everywhere, this eternal awareness is the heart. You play the game like everyone else, yet unlike everyone else, you are already there. It is because the Tantric Mandala of the Ascended Masters originates from this level, that it is already successful. It simply grows, awakening, one by one, in the reality of the Body of the One.

As you awaken into this awareness, you have always been awake. A twelfth-level adept has always been a twelfth-level adept. Time is not linear; it is a creation of the eternal.

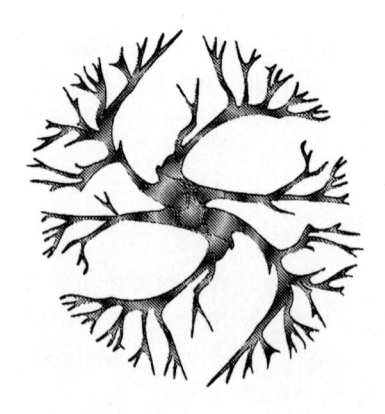

Developing a Body of Light

Earlier, I presented an initial understanding on bringing forth a subtle body of light above the head. In this chapter, further techniques will be given, pitfalls discussed, and various wisdoms presented. The subject matters addressed in this chapter are not in a one, two, three, do this then that format; rather, they are all various aspects necessary to be brought into a whole—various angles to be addressed and flavors that are pointed out. Together, they reinforce the same underlying transmission of how to progress within the Eternal Yoga practices.

Read this chapter every few months. Much of what is being said will have more relevance as you continue in your practice.

The purpose of words is to give enough knowledge, inspiration, and transmission to get things started. While book words are a start, and can be a subtle vehicle of connection with their author and/or truths, nothing replaces a living source of inspiration, guidance, and transmission. Yet, even with this, you must carry forth through your own practice into fulfillment. Through practice, you will discover what cannot be described in words.

Developing Definition

A key understanding for our yogic application is that consciousness and energy are two sides of the same coin. From the highest level of truth, consciousness is its own energy source.

Spirit is consciousness, forever radiating effortless energy, which we then clothe, that is—we modify the rays of our primal presence, repeatedly, into the various realms of our existence. As energy changes its characteristics, it becomes everything in creation, from a thought of love spread out across a vast vista of space to the rock at your feet.

Consciousness is always interacting with itself, forever changing its content. Nothing else exists in the entire universe, yet the whole universe is made of it. Eventually, we forget our original nature as primordial, fluid, consciously-conscious consciousness. This freezes our awareness into the relatively inanimate quality of its content, such as a rock, our identity as a human being, or even the wonders of an "individual" soul.

Whereas in the physical, we apparently get energy from what we eat, from exercise, or by absorbing cosmic energy from our environment—in the buddhic realms energy originates directly from consciousness, that is, it comes out of nothing that we would look upon in our world as tangible, such as food. Even if we were to experience eating a piece of cake in the buddhic realms, we know that this is an apparition made out of the thought "cake," being eaten by an apparition made out of the emanation we call "self." It is all consciousness interacting with itself.

In the physical, the degree of our consciousness waxes and wanes all the time. Sometimes we are very awake and aware, at other times, a truck could roll over us and we would not know it. Therefore, as we attempt to awake within more subtle realms, this awake/asleep type of awareness is not a good role model to base an understanding of how buddhic consciousness works. In the buddhic realms, there are also events that increase or decrease our level of awareness. However, if we know our spirit—the effortless source of energy, of consciousness itself, then we remain aware all the time. Thus, while we can use our existing awareness to initially support a more refined state of awareness, which we then further awaken within, and so on like rungs of a ladder—ultimately, only awareness as spirit is the full experience of that which never sleeps.

The equation of consciousness and energy works both ways. This is why yogis do breathing exercises to unite mind and breath. By extracting energy from the breath, we become more alive and conscious. We can use the two together, energy and consciousness, like alternate rungs of a ladder. By increasing our vitality, we use this as a support of consciousness and extend our awareness a bit further and a bit deeper. As we go deeper, we find that consciousness becomes its own source of energy.

As we attempt to go deeper in our meditations, many of us find ourselves eventually getting sleepy, lost in a formless space lacking the support of definition and energy. Consciousness, as awareness, is not some mechanical quality. Consciousness is consciousness because it is aware of something; it is something, not nothing. Thus, we need inner definition to stay awake.[1]

Footnote on next page

Developing character, standing for something, having opinions, developing approaches, knowing how to create something, being creative, are all vital for the spiritual path. We need definition to advance on the spiritual path. It gives our minds and energy something to focus upon, and in doing so we become more awake. As we become more awake, we have the opportunity to pay attention to the qualities of wakefulness itself and in this way, we get to know ourselves.

On the spiritual path, we extend this definition internally, so as to stay awake into a larger field of awareness, i.e., we are more than just a physical being. We need to learn how to strengthen our internal awareness by tangibly stabilizing it within a subtle form of prana. Internal visualization practices help us do this; for example, meditating as a letterform in the center of a chakra, or meditating as a tube of light-energy within our spine. This stabilizes our fickle mind by absorbing it into the subtle prana that we are visualizing, which results in bringing more tangibility to our subtle awareness. As we deepen, we learn new ways of defining ourselves. When you really understand this, then you can better understand why people do some of the things they do. You can understand, for example, why there are power maniacs[2]—because that is an approach, a method, of staying awake. As we deepen, we are also entering into a much greater transparency and thus, awareness of our co-creation of each other. Without this awareness, we are asleep; our ability to bring definition to ourselves in the higher planes is co-dependent with responsiveness to our transparent quality. Through acknowledging transparency, we develop sensitivity, refinement, and the

---

[1] There are further mechanics of getting sleepy while meditating. For example, the process of internalization often results in our consiousness shifting into the energy channels of the left side of the body. This is yogically corrected by purifying the channels of the left side and by bringing the left and right sides in balance—then entering, consciously, a deeper source. There is a distinction between getting sleepy because of the grosser, heavy pranas of the left side taking dominance and the sleepiness of not being able to follow the pranas into our central channel, as what often occurs in deep, restful, dreamless sleep. There is also the sleepiness of being absent and the sleepiness of low energy and identifying with that low energy state.

[2] There are those who thrive on the feeling of power (sensation) as an energy source. In this instance, control is secondary only to protect the availability of that feeling.

love required to develop our individuality—our definition—in the proper balance necessary for spiritual awakening.

It takes a lot of application and penetration to develop wakefulness on the subtle pranas of our existence. This is why we "practice." In essence, we are making the physical more transparent and the formless more tangible.

Practice this shift into transparency through the various activities of the day. Before eating some food, take a moment and inwardly lift that plate of food up to another realm. Have it blessed and see the food vibrant as light and energy. Make an offering of thanks and sharing by putting a little bit of the food on the ground for an animal or insect. Finding little ways to uplift energy, such as a smile or helpful gesture, is recognizing our transparency with each other. Transparency includes taking responsibility to keep your heart radiant and your thoughts uplifting. While growing up, I always thought that people could hear my thoughts and feelings, even a passing stranger. While I later realized that few people are this aware, it helped me to value my responsibility for my thoughts, and thus a motivation to remain clear within them. Even if people are not outwardly aware, on some level they are.

One of the best ways to increase definition is to breathe an awareness of light into your body. Learn to feel the various parts of the body. Sense your kidneys, liver, your dan-tien, your heart, etc. Feel and see yourself as a joyous being streaming forth nectar light. Vitalizing light and nectar within the body is perhaps the single most important activity we can do to increase our spiritual definition.

Another secret is shifting perspective within your practice. Perhaps for a few months you will focus mostly above the head and at other times, focus in a particular area of your body. Definition is multifaceted.

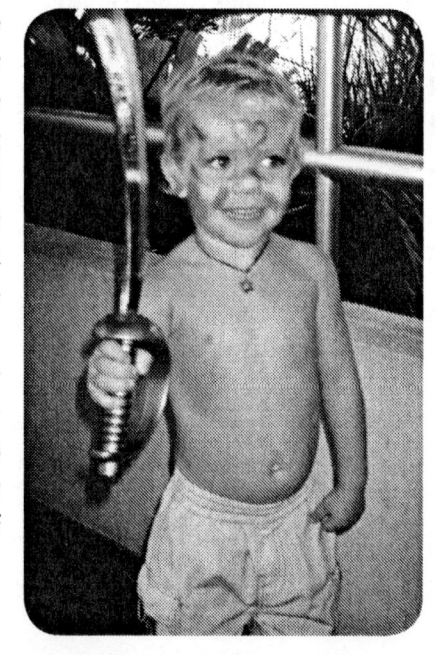

Symmetrical Awareness

By developing symmetrical awareness of our energy and presence, we can more easily see through distortions, purify them, and bring energy and awareness into our central channel.

Symmetrical awareness is a universal, innate truth, which yogis throughout the ages have understood. The principles of symmetrical awareness are easy to understand and apply. Simply, we are aware of the balance of energy on each side of our body and to a lesser degree, between the front and back. If our energy is primarily stuck on one side of the body, then this makes it difficult, if not impossible, to be aware from our center. Without awareness from the center, our energy does not enter the central channel. Without awareness in the central channel, we do not have the necessary refinement to enter into buddhic consciousness, which is the activation required to enter into the higher yogas, such as Eternal Yoga.

Habitually, most of us tend to live from and look to the phenomenal world, rather than reside within the stillness and depth of our center. As a result, the auric field of most people is always dancing out of balance. When we enter into yogic disciplines, it is a task to overcome this habit of looking left or right, of looking outward while forgetting the center. By becoming aware of where we are looking, in a tangible-spatial-feeling sense, we can energetically start to correct the imbalance, without having to get into the endless nitpicking details. This is a very direct approach to bring ourselves into a greater depth. An additional benefit is that we can realize immediate benefits to our health.

As transparent beings, we are always in some kind of cosmic participation. It is important to become aware of how we ground the cosmic connections of that cosmic participation into our body, in a tangible-spatial-3D sense. For example, feel a ray of light and connection extending from each shoulder into the cosmos. Make this about 30-degrees above horizontal. Similarly, feel a ray from each side of the top of the head extending out at about a 60-degree angle into the cosmos. Also, feel your central core and a line of awareness extending straight up. Is it just as easy to feel each side? This type of cosmic alignment is an important precursor to naturally awakening within buddhic awareness and in awakening above the head.

Since conscious communion and awareness of the Ascended Masters is so vital for the success of Eternal Yoga and the Tantras, two common questions are, "How do I know if I am really connecting with a Master," and "How can I discern if what I inwardly receive is distortion or truth?"

Before answering the above questions, it is important to understand there is no such thing as "connecting" to a consciousness that is outside of our selves. Thus, "our way of seeing" will always influence what we see and how we see. If we have a strong red disposition, then we will more easily see red. To see clearly, we need to know the delicate balance of blending from our core, i.e., the inherent nature of Oneness in which we all live.

The fullness of being able to do this requires our own movement into Mastery. There is a saying, "Only a Master can truly perceive a Master." Therefore, it all comes back to knowing ourselves in a pure light beyond the personality. In this way, we accept ourselves in the Ever-Expanding Perfection and our own growth within that. When you really know and accept that level of purity, then you know it. There is no mushy heart sentiment covering up what we do not want to see—it is very direct. There is a habit of taking every situation into ourselves, as a means of growth, within the Ever-Expanding Perfection. In this internal expansiveness, many words that would create a "Is this distortion or truth" scenario do not even come into play. Our purity brings us beyond that level of duality into the purity of presence. The way into that purity is often consistent practice, such as kriyas, of sufficient quality and quantity.

An inherent quality of the Masters is that they always have a strong, predominant presence within the central channel. This is how you can bring forth your awareness of the Masters in a pure way. For example, if you are ethereally talking with someone, bring that awareness into your central line. If you are focusing within the body, then this is your central core of prana. If you are focusing above the head, then this is a line of awareness that runs vertically straight up. If the energy insists in staying focused on one side or the other, then it is not sourced from the center. This is a quick and easy test. This distortion might be primarily from the being you are talking with, or from your side, or both. In truth, it is not important;

rather, if you cannot bring the focus into the central line, then why bother continuing? When you are in your center, then the presence is more important than the words. You are resting in radiant silence.

Bringing a telepathic relationship with another being into the central-line creates the equivalent of an eye-to-eye conversation. For example, by bringing a telepathic communication from some corner of your head to the front of your third eye and increasing the luminosity of the conversation, you can bring it from unconscious babble into a conscious interaction. This can sometimes involve a bit of inner-force, such as grabbing a mischievous energy and yanking it to your front. It is important that you are mature enough for this kind of activity, that you understand how not to be intrusive, unless necessary, and how to soften your energy with radiance, sensitivity, and humility.

Symmetrical awareness helps us to find our hidden sides and our weaknesses. It teaches us a lot about ourselves. It also keeps the importance of the body in perspective. Without bodily awareness, we do not have the anchor in which to perceive symmetrically. Understand that the consciousness within our central channel exists everywhere, yet it is a tremendously practical method to develop a focus of this as a central channel. In this way we can begin to feel that our body emanates from our core, and that this core is primal to the body, i.e., the body exists as a consciousness in the central core and emanates out from there.

All of the primal energy channels of our subtle body emanate into existence in pairs out of the central channel. There are myriad explorations and discoveries that you will find for yourself over the years. Remember the pair, both sides, whether it is male or female, solar or earth, introverted or extroverted, hot or cold, however you are relating. Then you can remain alive, blissful, and centered in the dance of creation.

So far, we have talked about two kinds of symmetrical awareness. The first was developing a balance within your energy field, so that you are naturally centered in the deepest core. It is only in this core that you will have the necessary depth of discrimination, based on a level of knowingness.

The second symmetrical awareness is about using the force of penetrating insight and the natural balance of purity to bring an energy front forward, rather than allowing it covertly, or ignorantly, to hide in the shadows. This forwardness also has a lot of intimacy, in that nothing remains hidden. Both of these methods are tools for deepening your energy and charting your way through the phenomenal fields of existence. These are very important for success in Eternal Yoga.

A third type of symmetrical awareness concerns opening the chakras. For example, it is a common visualization to become aware of sixteen filaments extending from the center of the throat chakra, horizontally extending out, and eventually branching into an endless network through the body. Extending awareness from the chakra, as light and feeling, through each of these filaments, will naturally create a balanced attentiveness and openness within the frequency of that chakra.

If you first create a basic balance within your body, you will have much more support to penetrate into and actually center within a chakra. Otherwise, your mind will most likely wander into something else. In regards to seeing the reasons for imbalance; some issues will show up more easily when working with the first and second type of symmetry, and some issues are easier to see in the process of establishing symmetry from within a chakra.

Continuing with our example of the throat center—suppose that normally, you find your attention is primarily on the left side of your throat. You sense that this occurs because of an imbalance deep within the throat itself. Therefore, you practice centering in the middle of your throat, embodying yourself there, looking outwards from that center instead of looking at it. Keep the area of focus small, this involves more subtlety and concentrates the energy, all of which helps you enter into the chakra itself. Then you might visualize yourself extending filaments of light simultaneously in all directions.

Commonly, for the throat chakra, this consists of sixteen filaments. I like to visualize the sixteen filaments, blue in color, all moving in a wave-like motion—like an octopus floating in inner space. It brings a feeling of beauty and energy. As you stay with it, you will feel a symmetrical balance occurring. All around the throat center will start to open up, and the two sides of the body will come into a greater balance. You will gradually energize your body as a whole. This is a way of working from the inside out.

Overcoming Doubt and Intellectuality

Without overcoming doubt, we cannot gain success in Eternal Yoga or the Tantras. Yet this is not something we can do by trying to boost our confidence; for example, through the emotional support of a religious group or the benefit of a strong faith. We only overcome doubt by direct experience. Yet, even after direct experience, some individuals are still plagued by doubt.

The awareness connected with through Eternal Yoga is not the same type of mind that you identify with through your thoughts. The higher-mind is transcendent, luminous, subtle, restful, and of a knowing nature which is formed by, and forms, the space of all that is encompassed by it.

Falling back into the old habitual, dualistic, way of thinking occurs, because this is your identity. This identity, your ego if you will, has a hard time accepting as real that which is outside of its identity. Even when a quiet inner knowingness knows the truth of this subtle mind, the outer mind still needs practice in letting go. Thus the solution is to keep at it—keep practicing, and keep moving forwards by letting go into that quiet knowing place within. You outer mind is not something you can talk to in this regards—it is like talking to a drunk; it simply does not understand within its framework. Rather, that inner, quiet, knowing place takes command, and repeatedly empowers your practice. This is something that you first learn how to do through creating your foundation, such as through the kriyas.

As you bring down this new awareness, again, and again, this light, which is after all, you, will start to break apart your old identity. It will create a new support structure into the physical. You will expand into a new awareness.

Enlightenment, while profound, is also very simple. Experiencing it once opens the gates to the long road of liberation; yet consciously residing within enlightened mind, to travel upon the road of liberation, requires cultivation. We need to become familiar with it. This cultivation starts with recognizing and valuing the simple beauty of the enlightened mind. This often takes many years, decades, even lifetimes on the spiritual path. Once we recognize what it is we are to value, we can purposefully employ skillful, mindful, and passionate ways to remain in this radiant simplicity.

Through remaining in enlightened mind, we grow into awareness of all the treasures that exist within its unlimited reach. Enlightened mind underlies everything, even the common mind[3] and its dualistic existence. While immersed in the immediacy of our limited identity, very few are able to identify the simple open radiance residing underneath this, without which nothing would even exist and thereby, remain in their true source.

Doubt results from the pulls of a limited mind, which cannot possibly see the bigger picture, and is thus simply expressing itself as such. Doubt is a lethal poison on the spiritual path because it has a way of keeping us wrapped up in this limited framework. If it were not for this limited framework, doubt would not exist. Furthermore, by trying to get rid of doubt through the activity of the common-mind, we go nowhere, as we are still in the activity of the common mind.

Do not lose heart that this is an almost impossible situation. There are clear and true ways to become free; this is what the tantric path is about. Eternal Yoga is that aspect of the tantric path that introduces us to the enlightened view, so we become fit and able to make our application, thus traveling the road of liberation in actuality.

Understand that this is a non-dual path. We get there by being there. Thus, to overcome doubt, deepen your practice beyond the framework in which doubt exists. Become more familiar with the effects of dissolving your dualistic awareness and all its prana into the heart. Doubt is simply part of the nature of duality. A dualistic mind cannot get rid of it, only temper it. You could use doubt, for example, by doubting the validity of what your elders say, and thus forging a new way. While this can have benefits or drawbacks on a social level, you are still in that limited mind. From the framework of liberation,

---

[3] Mind, in this instance is not referring to just our thoughts, but our life stream, thus it includes our thoughts, emotions, senses, etc.

the only solution is to deepen beyond it, anchoring yourself in that depth, then relaxing outwards again into an integrated continuum.

There are other ways that the effects of doubt and the dry fire of an overly intellectual mind are disastrous for the tantric path. In Tantra, we cultivate nectars within the chakras and the physical body, on which we embody the subtle mind. Doubt and excessive intellectuality are movements that draw the mind away from cultivating the nectars, which is a non-verbal process. It can dry them up so fast, that even with decades of attempted practice, tantric bliss is not experienced.

This is one of the reasons that periods of intensive retreat are so important. In these retreats, we do not read much or watch television and we do not apply ourselves to petty concerns of business or social niceties. We build the nectars. We devote enough time to become familiar with our true nature and effortlessly begin to reside within it.

When seriously plagued by doubt, stop and center yourself deep within your body. Feel your body turning into light. With each inhale, visualize the light of the body drawing into the center, and with each exhale, the light flowing out into the definition of the body. If you mind cannot let go of the issue in doubt, then simply breath it into the center as well, dissolve it, and as you breathe back out into the definition of your body, sense the perfection of your entire being instantly coming into existence. Know that you know beyond doubt. Meditate yourself beyond the unknowingness of doubt, to the knowingness of spirit.

Often doubt is a signal to relax a perspective. We may be trying to force something into a particular way of seeing, when what is required is a new angle. This kind of doubt is very healthy and part of the process of tantra, as the path of a thousand corrections. However, this is only effective if we trust ourselves and know that when we receive this signal: to relax, deepen, and discover. If we cannot quickly move in this way, then the healthy signal for change and deepening turns into confusion and a dull nature.

Doubt can be a judgment we make of our capacity. The solution is to deepen, relax, and discover. Our individual capacity in regards to a particular activity is something that we each discover, earn, and build upon, according to the particular purpose and passion of why we are here on Earth. This is a path of self-discovery. Doubt that surfaces in regards to an external application is not necessarily what we are addressing here; for example, "I doubt I could be the fastest runner in the world." The type of doubt being addressed is, "I cannot meditate," "I doubt the Ascended Masters, or my connection," or "I doubt I could enter into enlightened mind," or "I doubt I can overcome my self-created obstructions," even "I do not know if this is just my imagination or not." We all have a capacity to access the depth of own selves and through that, the infinite wisdom contained within the Body of the One. We must overcome this kind of doubt if we are to succeed on the spiritual path.

Three Modes of the Mind

I have observed three types of mind. Mind in this instance includes our emotions and awareness in general.

Most people reside their whole lives, with a few brief exceptions, within the common mind. It is thinking, acting and reacting, observing, feeling—while ignorant of ourselves as something beyond that.

A deeper level of mind is absorbing outer awareness into its source; for example, resting deep in the heart. It is non-verbal, the constant chitchat of the mind has stopped. In this kind of mind, we can still be conscious of the outer world, or perhaps not. When we are in this type of mind, we feel as if there are two worlds, the world ignorant of its source and the world aware of its source. They appear to have little in common with each other, other than a degree of awareness of primordial space existing through both.

In the third kind of mind, we are centered in our awareness as source, yet simultaneously "active" into all levels of existence, including an apparent use of the common mind. There is no separation. We feel everyone and everything as light emanating from source. In this state, we are inwardly and exquisitely very quiet and we are conscious of our thoughts and our existence as actively radiating out from this place through the love we feel, the thoughts we think, and the actions we do. There is no separation and there is no grasping, or trying to hang on to this state. We are both an individual and beyond individuality at the same time. This is the level of mind used in true teaching work from the level of the ascended body. It is not like the new-age concept of channeling at all. We experience this active state within the body literally as nectar that is silently and effortlessly radiating forth. Within this blissful-nectar, we can embody wisdom beyond our immediate individuality in an honest relationship with our personality to allow its empowered expression, and thus be in greater service.

A sufficient depth of nectar-consciousness includes an inherent awareness of primordial space. Within this activation, an active force of love skillfully reveals wisdom, directed by the inherent ever-expanding perfection into the exactness of its expression on many levels at once. Without this awareness of primordial space and of nectars within the body, there cannot be the true experience of this state of mind.

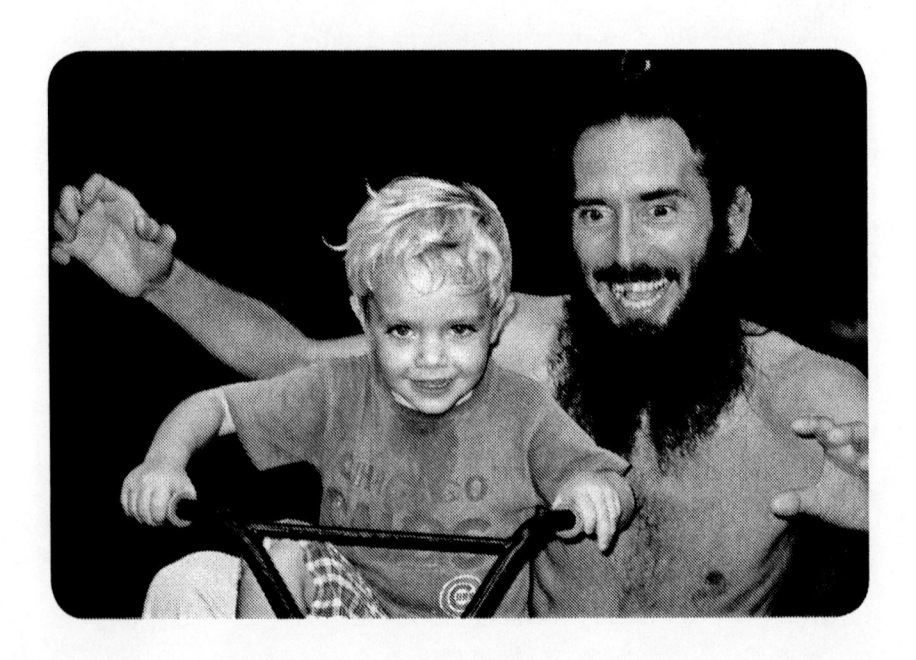

Becoming Comfortable with our True Nature

Many of the pitfalls addressed in this chapter have to do with a very subtle projection of ego-identification and grasping. This is different from a grosser display of egoic nature by a person with no activation into the subtle buddhic realms at all.

By purification through meditation, practices, and moving beyond the intellectualization or emotionalization of our conventional existence, we learn to rest in the simple spaciousness within our heart that is beyond grasping for identification. Simply resting in this depth can at first trigger an outer identity crisis. The ideas that we are so-and-so, or even that we are the experiences of our soul, all become empty, making way for the flowing radiance of spirit.

There is no immediate fix for this crisis. The willingness to go into these depths is the mark of those who are able to progress on the spiritual path. We must become comfortable with emptiness itself, with letting go of our minds and, even at times, our identity. We can only do this by becoming rich within and evolving enough to know or to trust that we do not exist because of our grasping, but by that which we already are, in the deepest of our natures.

In truth, even our souls are but temporary manifestations, ever-changing and blending. That which is forever is our spirit, and of this, there is no separation of spirit, one from the other; rather a dynamic display beyond the ability of the ego to understand. Spirit is consciousness and it is by this that we know ourselves beyond the outer identity.

While I constantly emphasize the importance of keeping meditation alive, to maintain the spark of awareness, this is not an excuse to avoid the difficult aspects of practice. Giving up the importance of our ambitions and perhaps not initially finding anything particularly exciting within can be difficult, especially when it involves giving priority to the loneliness of long meditation rather than the outer excitement of the world. This is a purification and a refinement.

It is important to meditate on the fact that without really understanding our true nature, we are like corks bobbing up and down in the endless sea of existence. Perhaps a higher experience here and a lower one there. We are not achieving liberation, just bobbing up and down on the swells of the endless ocean of experience, moving to the moods of others and our own desires. There is no way out of facing the truth of this, but, the more you embrace the lonely hours of dissolving the illusion, you will, by your own motivation, understand the depths and vastness of your true nature, which makes the world possible. There is no substitute for the hours of meditation required. It prepares the ground of realization by which we will succeed in the joy and light of our spirit.

It all depends on what you really want and your passion to achieve it. If you are willing, then you will go through what it takes. While it may sound cruel, even meditation and spiritual practices, without cutting to the core of our neurosis, just further bind us in illusion. It is a dangerous binding, in that we proudly think we have achieved something, yet we are just bobbing a little higher in the endless swells of the ocean. Practice serves to loosen the bounds of our identity, and through intensity, love, and the purity of our practice rightly directed, we dissolve into the spirited core-source of our being, finding endless joy within the beautiful flow of the Body of the One. In this gradual refinement, we non-verbally start to take notice of how our thoughts, our existence, even our soul, is but the clothing of that which is more than our individuality, yet is also us as an individual.

Projecting Limited Personality

By projecting into the empty space above the head, we develop awareness within that space, and thereby start the process of awakening within a very subtle body of light.

Because of our intention and initiation through the proceeding step of going far above the head, at least a portion of this projection will take root within the actual subtle dynamics of enlightened awareness. In time, more and more of our awareness within this subtle space originates from its own side and we awaken within buddhic awareness. Through maintaining a connection with the physical body, we develop an effortless continuum. Within the continuum we learn to distinguish which pranas are sourced from within the buddhic realms and which are secondary pranas originating from our more limited consciousness.

Problems arise when we start to look upon the projections of our limited consciousness as truths, rather than as a means. Because of the subtlety involved with the whole process, this is easy to do, particularly if we have a fascination with phenomenal activity and start to excessively search for it.

As long as you grasp at your identity and its experiences, and have not yet experienced the effortlessness of the Body of the One, you will be carried down the garden path of subtle or not-so-subtle illusions. The Ascended Masters often intensify this process by leading us into our karmas, not away from them. It may sound like an impossible scenario, the very thing we are using to help us awaken, is itself the danger. However, this is not a problem as long as the fires of purity, sincerity, and genuine practice stay alive. When these fires are well-established, the dynamics of the ego provides itself as fuel, thus purifying our self-perpetuated illusions.

If we choose to make our ego a god, rather than purifying it, then there is no end to the trouble we make for ourselves. This is a real danger, perhaps the greatest danger of the higher yogas and the one that has trapped many practitioners for eons. Ambition fuels this greatly, such as wanting what we are not ready for yet. Lust plays its part through the seduction of phenomena. Fear of the death of our limited self creates a covert existence. Too much fascination with power blinds us. Therefore, it is important that we remain diligent every step of the way.

A common example of projecting limited personality is the current channeling craze. While most of this is pure projection, occasionally some actually do channel another being or an aspect of their own higher self and are connecting into the buddhic realms. However, very few in this activity can distinguish between their personal colorings and those of with whom they are connecting. In addition, few understand the dynamics of the buddhic realms, including the distortions within them, let alone the lower realms that most people think of as the subtle realms. It is impossible to prevent one's personality from coloring what is "channeled," even if there is a genuine connection. The only solution is that one must know their self and have done the inner work. Those who truly know their self would most likely never enter into a channeling type of presentation, as this mode of presentation is too unclear in its implications and hype.

Another common example of projecting limited personality is hiding behind the phase, "Spirit told me so," or "God told me so," or similar phases. This is just too unclear. To illustrate, imagine the following analogy. Living in a large mansion, every morning you meditate in your favorite room. When you need answers to problems, or occasionally just to voice you musings, you speak into the universe. Amazingly, sometimes you here a voice in response, which you acknowledge as spirit or God talking to you.

Unbeknownst to you, in a room on the other side of the wall you are facing, there are a thousand people. Each of these people is an individual with their own opinions. When you speak, they hear your voice. Some pay attention, some do not. This particular morning, five answers come back and you hear one of them through the wall, which you qualify as, "God told me so."

To move past our analogy, often it is the various reaches of our own mind speaking to us. Our ambitions and biases often color the response we receive, even if it was a clear communication from a wise being. There is just not enough conscious recognition of what is going on, and as such, it makes it difficult to not only get a clear answer, but also to grow in consciousness itself.

A more conscious approach is recognizing the nature of oneness, and individualization as an expressive capacity of the oneness. You enter into the room, have a dialogue and communion, and then express your findings without losing the context that the content is inseparable from your own individual nature.

There are those pure of heart that can use this terminology of spirit and god as a path of the heart in relation to the divine. This purity of heart qualifies that they only, in this context of god, hear voices, receive vision, and feel presence from those of similar purity. A devotional nature can teach us the power of qualification and it keeps our focus on the divine. It can help us to transmute limited emotions into a greater love and emotion, opening up joy and happiness at even the hearing of God's name. A bhakti attitude can allow us to have introductory experiences of a state beyond words, for example, the Body of the One, or the glory of a particular Ascended Master. There is no need to say anything other than it is all God. This helps to the outer-mind out of the way. There are wonderful reasons to be on a bhakti path, and it is invaluable to experience it without reservation, at least for a time. Once truly entered, it is never lost. However, there are also disadvantages of a pure bhakti path. A pure bhakti path is not one of discrimination. It tends to fall apart when attempting to open up areas particularly resistant to penetration, such as a deep hurt that does not want to be seen, because the practitioner will often simply mask or avoid the issue. It also does not work for our application of Eternal Yoga as it keeps us ignorant and blind through a lack of penetration and internal definition, particularly within the buddhic realms. This transition from bhakti to discriminatory awakening can be a dangerous one if the ego gets the upper hand, so a teacher is of great help at this time.

Bhakti is the sparkling of divine love, the reaching up to love, the becoming of love, and the expression of love as all there is. As already emphasized, once known, it is never forgotten. In our spiritual journey, this bhakti is the divine spark, the joy of the nectars, the merging of the impersonal and the personal, the love of the Masters and the fuel behind our spiritual journey. In Eternal Yoga, we do not allow ourselves to hide behind a self-created "cloak" of unenlightened-bhakti. This cloak is a common way of covertly projecting subtle personality, without holding itself accountable. We are warriors who are not afraid of definition and we cut through unconsciousness. While enjoying the softness of love—we embrace bliss, free ourselves of delusions and fearlessly expand our hearts in cosmic awareness. We elevate our presence to become deeply radiant and enjoyable, while penetrating and beckoning divine discovery for all those who come across it. This is true bhakti.

One of the most dangerous, and somewhat unavoidable, projections of semi-enlightened consciousness is participation within a group mind of similar semi-enlightened beings. Here there is an underlying shared motivation to maintain particular blind spots and common ambitions of power and influence that are ignorantly or purposely not in alignment-awareness of the Body of the One. Of course, such a mindset would never word it in this way, or even acknowledge it. It often creates a form of resistance that is subtly clever. This support continues even into very subtle levels of buddhic mind space of this group consciousness. The highest fruit of this path is liberation into the illusory self, rather than liberation from the space of pure spirit. It is entering into the realms of the gods.

Each of us have participated in and have gained definition through various star cultures. For example, Pleiades, Sirius, Arcturies, Antaries, Orion... There are also collective states of consciousness created through an inner attunement independent of an outer location. To aid in the definition of the culture and its spiritual advancement, collective supports are established by and for its participants. Yet, in the whole mandala of our being, no part is complete without the whole. Each particular facet, on its own, has its limitations. When our sole frame of reference and support is a particular school, we become bound within those limitations.

As an example, perhaps because it is a troublesome and widespread example, from a planetary perspective, are the Arcturians. Many souls who have maintained a close identity with their Arcturian culture enjoy some of its cultural understandings, which include a subtle identity within the eighth and ninth realms. This serves as an activating principle to propel many of its members into a semi-enlightened awareness within these realms, yet the lack of spiritual preparation often results in disaster. A lack of spiritual work may result in a mental quality of this awareness running away with itself compounded by a very arrogant disposition. These projections have extended into sacred places of the earth, into power plays, politics, and delusions on a grand scale. It can bind its participants in a self-perpetuating play for eons. For these souls, the only way out is to break the bubble and release themselves from this identity, deepening their spark of aliveness. Then, when they have the proper development, they can go back to work and play within these cultures, if desired.

While the above has been used as a particular example, each of us must, as we are spiritually ready, break free from the cultures of our upbringing: poor, middle class, rich, earth-based culture, city-based culture, star-based culture, religious, atheist, an eclectic mix, it does not matter. This breaking free is not necessarily a rebellion or a lack of respect, rather, it is to know ourselves on a deeper level and gain identity from that. Breaking free of cultural identity without spiritually finding ourselves is of little use and most likely will result in aimless wandering.

The Spark of Aliveness

There are various ways that we project un-enlightened or semi-enlightened existence through buddhic space. As pertaining to development within Eternal Yoga, the first of these is our everyday-physical, or physical-like awareness that we subtly project as a means to staying awake.

As we awaken into effortless awareness originating from the realms above the head, we will experience a mix of buddhic consciousness and that which we are projecting from below. It is advantageous to maintain awareness of the body so that we can more easily identify the components of this mix. We can also use bodily awareness as an aspect of this continuum to provide the polarity in which to become aware of areas we need to see about ourselves and as a way of gaining symmetrical perspective. Bodily awareness enables us to advance upon the path of Eternal Yoga into the Tantras, as we will have automatically deepened into the central channel and will instinctually understand the yoga of nectars (when the time comes to apply ourselves in this way).

The danger of this mix is that we are supporting it from limited consciousness, rather than the purity of spirit. This is why it is so very important to connect to that point way above the head and to mature this into the depth of the heart. This is why an infallible connection to an Ascended Master is necessary. If you do not return to the simplicity of your true nature, then you will become lost. Without being able to distinguish the difference between buddhic-light-body awareness lacking a vibrant awareness of spirit as source, and awareness originating in spirit, from the perspective of Eternal Yoga, we are lost.

When firmly anchored in spirit awareness, the vista is much vaster and unmistakable. You are in the Body of the One, and while existing as an individual, strongly so, you have in fact, ceased to exist solely as an individual. When not anchored in this, it is difficult to distinguish between the two. To the ignorance of the outer world, you can appear as a very advanced practitioner. You can be a siddha, have a lot of projection, and say nice words. You can wow people with subtle projections and have many stories to tell. You can enjoy sublime states. Yet in truth, you are deluded, still caught in a subtle binding of limited personality that does not know how to escape. You may not even be aware of your predicament. This is one of the reasons that a competent teacher is so important.

The spark of aliveness is just that—a spark. Always find the spark of aliveness in your practice. Simplicity and bliss, humbleness and definition, focus and relaxation, individuality and oneness, effort and effortlessness, purity and acceptance—when we can bring these pairs together, we are naturally in a correct mode of spiritual awareness by which we can get there by being there.

Visualizing a Body of Light above the Head

One of the key practices of Eternal Yoga is bringing forth a body of light above our head as a vehicle of enlightened-consciousness.

There are two approaches to bringing forth a radiant identity of light as an enlightened activity. One is meditating upon the image of an already enlightened Master and becoming that image. The other is to awaken our own image, as we already know it through our physical body, into light. Both are powerful methods, each with certain advantages and disadvantages. As either practice eventually matures into an awareness of the Body of the One, it is principally a difference in how we start the process rolling. As this maturity occurs, you will use both approaches in a natural understanding of how to work within the Body of the One.

As a technical note: it is not strictly necessary to create a particular image in the buddhic realms to have consciousness in those realms, as we can simply embody upon the particular scenes and pranas of which we are momentarily aware. For example, you might spontaneously become aware of a field of light and sensation, a sacred understanding, the image of a friend, a whole town in all its details, or simply the sensation that your physical world is a projection from a deeper aspect of yourself. However, by creating an active light-body, you are better able to stabilize your awareness. This light body becomes a template for your physical body, and as the two merge, you can extend your ascension into the physical.

Visualizing Yourself above the Head

Within the Eternal Yoga practices, this is the approach appropriate for most people to start with. You begin by visualizing your own image above the head.

There is a combination of effort, and within that effort, an effortless discovery of your own buddhic nature. For some, this discovery comes quickly, often because of activity from previous lives; for others, they have to work at it more.

To start with, first get in touch with your own body. Kriyas, conscious breathing, and exercise all help to increase vitality and thus awareness of ourselves. Visualize and feel your own body exactly as it currently is. As you get in touch with this, then feel that you are sitting above your head with this same image. It is as if you have two bodies. If there is a favorite activity that comes to mind, sometimes visualize yourself doing this activity.

Some people have an easier start with visualization. Some have an easier start with feeling their presence and then stabilizing that feeling presence, as if you can see by the sense of feeling. The reason for using an image of you, rather than simply a sphere of light, is that you are increasing self-definition. Definition within the light is what helps us to become awake, and allows us to re-define ourselves within our spiritual growth.

Bring as much light and transparency as possible. Our principal responsibility to ourselves, and to others, is to become a radiant being, joyful to experience. This is an inner condition we are cultivating, not an outer mask. Find the nectars of your existence and cultivate them for the benefit of yourself and all beings. At some point, you will start to spontaneously transition from a projection of this image above your head to an effortless emanation of it from within the buddhic realms.

Spontaneously experiencing yourself as a divine image in the buddhic realms requires a degree of activation. For the sincere practitioner who has done the preliminary work, this transmission can be self-initiated. This is one of the gifts of Eternal Yoga.

Spiritual transmission occurs through the common ground of oneness. It is a consciousness of activation. You have to be willing to feel and to become what you are receiving. To give you an idea how transmission occurs, suppose you want to develop a greater feeling of strength. Through your intention, you come into the company of a person who exudes a wonderful sense of strength. Just being in this person's presence helps you to feel stronger. No words are necessary. Possibly, before you set this intention, you may not have particularly noticed this person. After a while, you can say to yourself, "Now I know what strength feels like. I will further cultivate my own image into this feeling and thereby gain my own strength." You have received from this person the transmission of what strength feels like.

In the process of self-initiation, we open ourselves to a greater possibility. We feel, visualize, and identify ourselves as a divine sparkling of transparent light, naturally, directly, and intimately. In the acceptance of that divinity, we are opening ourselves to other divine beings and previously hidden aspects of our own self that can help us further in this feeling and awareness. As we truly open up, it is impossible not to become aware of an activating presence, even if we have no name or words for it. We enter into an inner space literally made out of the consciousness of those who are awake within it—the Oneness.

In receiving higher transmission, there is a sense of being meditated upon. While you have made the effort, suddenly you are just experiencing this activity occurring. All you have to do is be aware of it. You know that, from your more limited framework, it is not you doing it, so why the emphasis on self-initiation? Because, without taking a degree of responsibility in your part of the equation, of how you have called this forth, then you will not be in an empowered place to make the application required of what you have received. Using our previous example, getting an initial feeling of strength is not enough. To make it yours, you have to cultivate your own image of this feeling. If you want liberation, you will have to apply yourself towards it.

Sadly, many believe that transmission is something that occurs beyond their level of understanding. If a teacher taps them on the head with a flower or sprinkles some holy water on them, that this is all the transmission requires. They fumble for years, holding onto this belief structure, never having the necessary level of activation (direct awareness). As a result, they go nowhere.

There are those who already have the necessary vision of where they are going, but do not believe they are qualified to practice until they get that sprinkle of water, possibly ignoring the true transmission they already have in favor of a mental construction bound to a static set of belief structures. Self-initiation bypasses many outer belief structures and shifts the emphasis to accepting self-responsibility for directly refining our own inner belief structures. This is the attitude needed for success within Eternal Yoga.

While transmission itself occurs effortlessly, we have to work towards the space in which it occurs. We are changing ourselves, opening and molding our consciousness to a new possibility. You earn what you keep by demonstrating your willingness to play in the bigger picture that you are invoking. Along with consciousness comes responsibility in how you hold that consciousness.

Do not let the concept of self-initiation lessen the importance of a teacher or the transmissions obtained from within that relationship. You must take responsibility for "consciously" entering into a level of activity, and calling that forth. No teacher or divine being can do this step for you. Even if a Master is activating and working with your buddhic self, if you do not open yourself to perceiving this level of activation, then you still sleep. You must actively apply yourself. You have to get past any images or thoughts that keep you bound in a limited perception, and you reflect, "I Am this activity." Then you actively deepen yourself to perceive it for yourself.

Initiation seldom occurs all at once. While each step may be profound, a full awareness of the bigger picture takes time to obtain. What we bring forth with self-initiation is the possibility itself of opening the doors to our own true nature. A spiritual teacher can work with us to greatly accelerate the process, and share transmissions with us beyond any conceivable measure of outer value. A teacher can also ignite within us the desire to awaken from a long sleep.

Some practitioners have a hard time accepting themselves as divine beings. The everyday mind and emotions become overwhelming and end up spoiling the whole thing. If you find yourself in this predicament, you may need more kriya practice, yoga, and general spiritual growth. There are preliminary preparations necessary for the Eternal Yoga practices to bear fruit.

There are additional advantages to using your own image as a vehicle of buddhic awareness. Some of these are:

> *1) In the process of generating a self-image, you have to connect to your body as an image of light. This is a purification and refinement in its own right. You will learn more about yourself in this process.*
>
> *2) A projection of your own image makes it easier to stay awake in the process, as you can always use the pranas of your physical body to aid in this projection.*
>
> *3) Mentally constructing what a particular deity looks and feels like for some makes the whole process too mental and dry. It is often easier to start with something that is very familiar to you, i.e., your own image and presence.*
>
> *4) An important principle of Eternal Yoga is maintaining simultaneous awareness within our physical body and the buddhic realms. It is awareness of the two that allows us to see our seed-karmas in a framework of the Ever-Expanding Perfection. Using an image of ourselves, as we currently are, helps greatly in this simultaneous awareness, as the reflection of your seed-karmas into physical realities are more easily recognized. In short, we have a better opportunity to see our blind spots. It is very honest.*

5) You will discover and emphasize the qualities that you bring to the light. You will more easily obtain a dynamic understanding of how you are part of the light.

There are some disadvantages of starting out with your own image above your head. A competent teacher can help you to avoid these potential pitfalls. Some of these pitfalls include:

1) You might confuse the pranas that your personality uses to help support everyday consciousness with the buddhic nature itself. While this is also possible using a mental construct of a deity, in the process of using your own image it is easier to egoicly think you have achieved a level of spiritual advancement, when you actually have not yet achieved anything of spiritual significance.

2) You might start cultivating a subtle level of inappropriate egoic projection. You may start using your newfound playing field to get what you want from a level of personality. This often results in huge amounts of delusion. To some degree, this is unavoidable, but if it gets out of hand, this is a serious problem with far-reaching consequences. Remember to keep the purity. Maintaining a level of feminine sensitivity is often the way to move within buddhic space. This includes responsibility for maintaining an uplifting presence that is joyous and opens up a sense of space. There is an art to blending with others that must be learned, requiring a humbleness, honesty, and awareness.

The bulk of practice within Eternal Yoga involves itself with this image above your head. It is paramount to remember that achieving this definition, by itself, is not enough and can become a vehicle for spiritual entrapment. You need to develop this definition within the context of the radiant purity of your spirit.

This includes keeping everything in a context of spiritual development. There is a lot of advertising that occurs in these realms.

There are righteous causes and belief structures. Remember, we either bind or free ourselves within these realms. If we keep a level of purity, then we will be able to further apply ourselves, successfully, within the tantras and achieve full liberation. Purity in this context refers to valuing the radiance of spirit itself. This radiance, which lies behind the mind, gives us the ability to cut through the subtle levels of the mind.

While you need self-definition to awaken, it is radiant awareness itself that is the key, not the content of your awareness. In the process of discovery, if you lose yourself for the content, rather than remaining in the purity of radiant-awareness itself, then you have simply expanded the playground of delusion and have lost the plot.

It all comes back to keeping awareness of the divine spark alive. In the words of Paramhansa Yogananda, "Love is the beginning, the middle, and the end."

Visualizing Ourselves as an Ascended Master

In this approach, you bring forth the image of one of the Ascended Masters above your head and imagine that you are that being. If successful, you essentially become that being, and thereby experience the enlightened qualities of that Master. For most practitioners, I believe it is better to start the process of buddhic activation using their own image. There are exceptions to this, as will be described further in this section.

Upon emphasizing that we use our own form as the subject of our visualization above the head, please do not take this to indicate that we should not develop a relationship with the Ascended Masters. This emphasis of using your own image is the primary focus. Within that focus, there will be a lot of variation, and occasionally your focus itself is entirely different. It is not always you doing it; at times, the Masters themselves will be meditating you. This also includes your highest self,[4] meditating you into awakening.

---

[4] Some people will claim the subtle voices of ego to be their enlightened self. Be careful, keep the spark alive, and let the content flow in context.

Developing a Body of Light   103

There are many discoveries to make. For example, some practitioners will give their image such a sun-like quality that they are not able to blend. Other people may then experience you as an overbearing quality. In that case, there will come a time requiring a more feminine, soft, and water-like quality. The same applies, in reverse circumstance, for someone who is so soft in their essence, that they need the sun-like quality to come into balance.

In the later stages of practice, as we blend within the Body of the One, we will often experience ourselves through the forms of various Masters,[5] and the whole discussion of which method to start with (our own image or that of a deity) becomes mute.

Most of the higher Buddhist Tantras will have you begin the process of activation by visualizing yourself as a deity, such as the inwardly or outwardly given representation of an Ascended Master who allows one of their forms[6] to be in service in this capacity. There are some wonderful advantages to starting with this approach. If these reasons, such as in the following paragraphs, apply to you, then you may want to start with this approach instead. Remember, as you progress, eventually both approaches lead to the same result, as long as you are able to actually progress and do not get stuck along the way. Another reason to start with this approach is if you are under a competent teacher who uses this method and can guide you in the details.[7]

---

[5] Of course, we do not only blend with Masters, but with all life itself, enlightened or not. What is being addressed is a focused application specific to the purpose of greater buddhic awakening.

[6] Not all deities are the direct presence of a particular Ascended Master. Sometimes a Master will develop an image and associated activity, then release that soul-image for use by a number of Masters and Adepts. In addition, not all deities originate from the level of the Ascended Masters, but sometimes from adepts who are close to that level of achievement.

[7] If you have a relationship with a competent teacher that brings forth a pure level of transmission, then that is everything. It is important to understand that various teachers use methods that are not so much empowered by the outer facts of the techniques, but by an inner resonance with the teacher themselves, opened up through the practice. The teacher will use this as a vehicle of further transmission that cannot be understood through any book. This is a very sacred relationship. If you are fortunate to be in this kind of relationship, then leave your mind out of it and practice with sincerity. Keep the spark of direct awareness alive.

Identifying yourself as another form, may help you to release a habitual grasping of identity. It can alter the way in which you see the world, resulting in enlightenment. If you truly have a connection with the deity you are visualizing, then you will be able to sense the quality of buddhic activation, and thus become initiated into this awareness. When properly meditating upon, with, and as a deity, you can use the power of devotion to help focus your pranas. Through the activation of this love, you can experience a direct connection with the already realized subtle body of the deity, and thus experience for yourself the nature of buddhic consciousness.

For this to occur, you must have a true connection with the deity. For example, you may always have felt the presence of Jesus or Krishna with you. You may get the connection again in a dream, or receive it through feeling it in another, such as your teacher. There are many ways.

By merging in this way, you may experience directly what the Body of the One feels like. There are many, many reasons that this approach can bear great and quick fruit. So why should everyone not start in this way?

In reality, we only gain such fruit when we are consciously residing in that pristine clarity ourselves. Subtly, our personality will color everything. This type of pristine clarity is not something we can achieve by the mechanical exactness of a particular way of meditating. It entails our involvement with many beings, the images we have imprinted within the earth, the blissful creation of destinies we have created within our soul, and thus, the very alive discovery of ourselves in an incredible richness. It is a long work in progress, and along the way we forget and lose the divine view, settling within apparent separation and its rules of engagement. We become afraid of moving beyond separation, less we lose our identity, and we even forget that separation itself has perfection within it, a divine reason for being.

There is a lot of subtle and not so subtle personality that has a force behind it born from the necessity of survival in the only way we have managed, so far, to stay somewhat awake. This is what the ego is. While we might seek relief by simply chucking it all out the door, by meditating ourselves as some other already radiant and enlightened being, most of us will just end up hiding aspects of our egoic personality behind this image, making it more difficult to see. While some argue that we are transforming these traits, and there can be a great truth in this, experience shows that for most of us, it is not so simple. We have to recognize our light, our energy, our presence, and our own Ever-Expanding Perfection. We have to first unravel the confusion we have created, by finding our own image in a divine light. If we will self-initiate this step, we will receive help from those who have gone before us. Then we can begin to understand ourselves in a larger context. Through this self-definition, we blend into the greater body of oneness and find true peace. This is the difference between gaining mastery and forever remaining in a level of blindness to our own divinity.

As we activate our own image, clean house, and discover ourselves from, and eventually beyond, the light, we automatically awaken beyond our individuality. We will simultaneously be aware of our image and those who we blend with, all in recognition of the underlying ground of oneness.

For some, there are compelling reasons to again ignite the buddhic activation primarily through identification as a particular Ascended Master. The Master will meditate you into this relationship, as an emanation. There is already a soul-likeness in which the connection can actively occur. In this circumstance, however you start, as you begin to apply yourself, you will find yourself in this practice. It is rare, and inherently understood by the practitioner beyond any need of explanation. Such a practitioner is simply carrying forth the work from a previous lifetime, and as such, is getting a kick-start, and even then, only when the timing is right. This timing often involves maturation through preliminaries involving the same kind of kriya practice and life experience by which we all progress.

In regards to the increasingly popular so-called higher tantric teachings of identifying yourself totally as a deity, given to anyone willing to study, pay an event fee and accept a so-called empowerment, this is a gross misrepresentation of these teachings and as such, results in a greatly compromised situation for most who are entering into these teachings. The atmosphere, while perhaps enriched in some ways, is often lacking of any real tantric flavor, even if the teacher has some inner understanding of it, and the transmission simply does not flow under the contrived conditions. The underlying blockages and emotions practically screaming to be addressed are usually ignored, suffocated under false concepts of what the tantric path is. This includes the agendas of those trying to keep their priesthood alive and well, seemingly oblivious to the basic understanding that the tantras only flourish in those who are not bound to a mindset of social conditioning. To move energy, we must be able to embrace change, including changing our own nature. With all this, there is sincerity within these events, and somehow some growth does occur, but often people get stuck again.[8]

Despite being presented otherwise, these practices are not so much a tantric activation into buddhic awareness, but a kind of transformational kriya, often with no buddhic activation occurring at all. If in this context, we recognize these techniques as a type of kriya instead of a tantra,[9] the practitioner will not be mislead by ideals they are not ready for yet, and can more honestly practice and thus gain fruit. Tantra requires that we are able to go beyond the mind. It starts from the highest levels into a practical realization of

---

[8] I am addressing the current means of teaching within the western world of the Tibetan Tantras. Of course, there are some very dedicated and remarkable teachers within this lineage. A few have gained great benefit and many have gained some benefit from these teachings.

From my vantage point, I have observed that, for the most part, the inner essence of the teachings is dying within this format. This is a shame, because there is a body of practitioners who could make a difference in cutting through all the widespread distortions so prevalent in today's spiritual atmosphere. Instead, for the most part, they are caught within their own bubble of grasping at the outer form of the religion.

If the precious radiations are going to survive, then they will need to be opened up through the enlightened essence of truth to address the conditions of those whom they are being presented to, without deluding the passion of what is required to succeed. Many think that the way of preventing this deluding of content is to stick to translating scriptures; however, this is simply making them dead. What is of value is the living presence of nectar. This requires an enlightened presence dynamically helping others to uncover this enlightened essence for themselves.

If the dharma is not to become a cult in America, then it will have to overcome its patriarchal prejudice and openly embrace and become once again empowered by the feminine origin and wisdom of the tantras, presenting a balanced spiritual approach. It is the axis beyond form, by which the Twin Ray descends into manifestation that is both how the tantric schools are overseen as a means of liberation, and as the hope of transformation itself on this planet.

the continuum. If you are not yet able to, or willing to go beyond your mind, then you will simply put your mind into endless contortions and delusions. At this stage, kriya, or similar approaches, is your path.

Occasionally, there is a person receiving these teaching who is able to take them as a tantric practice, as they are already in the enlightened state necessary in which to start. Such a practitioner will take this enlightened state into further buddhic activation and then quickly open into our true nature originating as radiant awareness—resulting in full enlightenment and recognizing that, in essence, you have always been there—it is just that you were not aware of it. You are able to begin the journey of liberation, otherwise known as ascension, for you will get there because you are, in awakened essence, already there.

The practice next advances into the development of this continuum through further development of our enlightened core within the body and then its flowering within the earth, the sphere of compassionate influence, and the immediate individual bodily presence as well—all occurring in a roughly simultaneous display of the Ever-Expanding Perfection that cannot outwardly be understood. All this has the sweetness and frequent personal enjoyment of simplicity, beyond constraints of the mind. In the tantric ideal of this practice, you "begin" by opening the top of your head and your heart (as well as your whole body) and feel yourself "as" the Deity, which you already

---

[9] The difference of a particular practice being a kriya or a tantra lies largely in the level of realization of the practitioner. An enlightened practitioner can use what outwardly appears as a kriya practice, in a tantric context. An un-enlightened practitioner, will at best be practicing a tantric teaching as a kriya, and at worse, just be muddling in confusion and creating confusion in others as well. Practices such as Eternal Yoga, when properly entered, are the initiatory aspects of tantra, whereby we gain the proper view in which to further progress in the tantras.

Seducing ourselves into the apparent freedom and phenomenal pull of tantra, without being ready, simply results in a lot of projection and psychic pollution. The self-responsible application towards radiance through kriya and general spiritual purification, including alignment with Mother Earth, is what is first required. Try to understand what is being said under the semantics. Misunderstanding of the various aspects of spiritual practice has resulted in a lot of confusion, essentially resulting in a wrong use of tools for the job at hand. This has largely resulted because many teach who themselves have no idea of the larger picture, and because it is simply an extension of confusion keeping things confused, so that nothing really changes. Effective spiritual practice changes everything.

feel identified with—and have never really been separate from. It is an active quality. Your identity literally becomes this and is felt as a presence emanating out from within the nectars of your being, and also as a subtle overlay of your physical body from within and around every cell, as an identification and a radiance. Cosmic fires are delightfully consuming you— yet from the ego's viewpoint, they are terrifying. You willingly ask for more, having tasted reality. You as an individual are dying, you no longer exist just as an individual. It is not just your identity that is changing, but how you see every identity. The whole concept of identity itself is being transformed. Your worldview changes and it is only Love that keeps you here and intact. Without the bliss of love, without the Masters, you do not exist at all. Yet the degree that you can be of Love, honestly within the nature of the Body of the One, still hinges on how well "you know your own self." This is not a mental idealization. You will become liberated—or else you will very much know that you are lost, which is a kind of insanity. You will grasp, for the time being, back into a limited identity, knowing that there is perfection in separation that prepares us through individual definition. Few have the passion, penetration, and loving-grace to enter such a tantra so directly. There are decades and lifetimes of preparation. Most are kidding themselves. You have to know yourself first! Yet the fullness is open to each and every one who sincerely applies themselves towards it, with the constant prayer of the greatest good for all beings.

For most of us, we must first start with where we are, and use this to help unite our body, breath, and mind in a nonverbal wholeness where we become fit to enter the larger spiritual discovery. While challenging at times, this is enjoyable.

The following example illustrates how, even if presented as a tantric practice, kriya is still the predominant mode of practice for most sincere practitioners, as it should be. In a typical meditation, as given through the generation stage of Buddhist tantric practice, you work in meticulous detail to bring forth all the aspects of your visualization, such as the principal deity and other deities, a courtyard, flowers, etc. You gain a greater capacity and you become absorbed into this focus, and through further refinement, you learn how to absorb the pranas inwardly through the initiation of this focus.

Through the subject of your focus, you transform the scope of your identity, and release yourself into the necessary transparency. In short, you are preparing yourself to be able to see what is already present. This is kriya, which works with a principal of transformation. In contrast, Tantra starts from the viewpoint of enlightenment.

As we continue, if we honestly do the work, we may release our grasping mind enough to notice the already present enlightened ground in which we inherently stand. In this way, we may actually notice the true nature of the deity we are meditating upon, allowing that deity to in turn meditate us, and help us, for that moment, to truly begin the tantric path. Yet, as we become more intimate, that being will only serve to return us to ourselves, and once again, we are on a path of purification and self-discovery. We are back to kriya and all the ins and outs of spiritual growth as it applies to us as an individual. Step by step, we will make it. There is a profound wisdom in saying that for most people, it is best to start with their own image and self-initiate it into buddhic awareness, for these steps are inherently recognized as part of the process. It is a smoother transition from the kriyas into the enlightened view of the tantras, which is the aim of Eternal Yoga.

To demonstrate a typical problem that results in meditating oneself as a deity before one is ready for it, quite a few times, I have seen various practitioners in my meditation or dreams, cloaked in the body of the being they are attempting to identify with. They will come looking just like a figure from a painting, of course a bit more life-like. So, while so-and-so will come looking like a popularized image of Padmasambhava, for example, there is a world of difference between the actual and full presence of Padmasambhava and this projection. These practitioners have simply replaced a grosser level of grasping at their immediate form with grasping at an idealized form. Because I know and have had countless interactions with Padmasambhava himself, I can positively state the rather obvious difference. In contrast, a master such as El Morya can come in the form of Padmasambhava for a particular purpose, and there is no incongruity at all. Padmasambhava himself can blend with many forms; he can appear as and embody through all sorts of beings, yet the buddhic mastery and clarity that he is remains unmistakable.

At times, he is in every cell of my being, he is seeing through my eyes, and talking through my mouth. There is a total blending, and within this, I know who I am (which is not separate) and there is no confusion whatsoever. Blending within the Body of the One is very natural, effortless, and fluid. You remain yourself and can become the universe at the same time. It is beyond that which words can describe.

It is the direct awareness of primal radiance that we are releasing our habitual focus into noticing. This is the aim of Eternal Yoga. It is only from this place of consciousness that we can effortlessly blend within the Body of the One, and in so doing, we expand in the Ever-Expanding Perfection of our true nature. How you see everything is changed.

Rather than a contrived connection to a deity, through so-called tantric visualizations of what the Master looks like, in the more feminine and direct approach, the whole success results from an instantaneous sense of connection; you simply feel through an open heart. This is the way of the Body of the One.

It is no different from feeling the presence of a loved one, such as a child or your lover. You can claim no great spiritual ability in simply feeling a family member. Everyone has this ability. We are simply expanding this to a greater depth. In a mature connection within the awakened Body of the One, there is a feeling of family from the start, and you have all the benefits and naturalness of a family affair.

The details fill themselves in spontaneously and as needed. You may not know what El Morya looks like, but you are aware of his presence and that is enough. This is more important than meditating on a contrived appearance as an attempt to get a connection. This approach is the one naturally entered into through Eternal Yoga. It requires that you are clear, activated into buddhic awareness, and that you know your true nature. Start with your own image, know the trappings, and keep the spark alive.

The Higher Realms within the Earth

Awakening within the inner realms of the earth and discovering our images in these realms is an important part of growth. The images we hold within the earth are like film in front of a projector. As the light shines through the film (the images in the earth), this results in a projection of these images as an etheric blueprint helping to create the ins and outs of our daily life.

Getting in touch with this not only helps us to be more aware, but also we have the opportunity to change. While this is not the subject of this particular book, awakening within the buddhic realms gives us the necessary depth to see within the inner realms of the earth. This is of a much deeper nature than the surface realms most shamans explore. It is a mistake to think of the buddhic realms as something beyond the earth. To paraphrase, as you awaken above the head, you also have the ability to awaken much deeper within the earth.

A Final Point to Remember

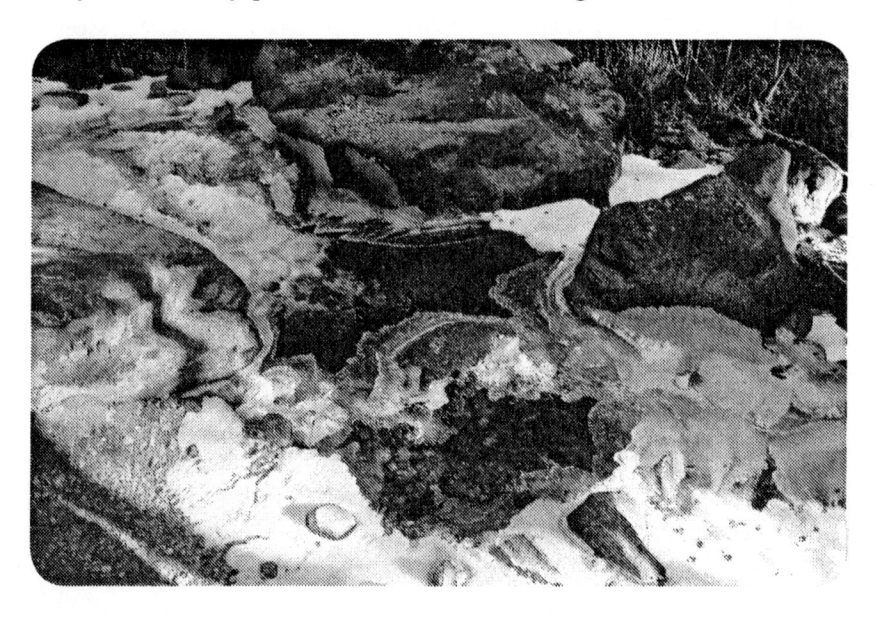

In reality, the buddhic realms do not exist just above your head. They are in every point of creation. Accessing them above the head is a potent and extremely practical physiological and psychological short-cut method of becoming aware of these realms.

As a psychological relationship, going above the head automatically puts us into a framework not immediately supported by our everyday consciousness. We remove ourselves from a level of personality. Going further above the head further increases this level of transcendence. Going above the head gives us a working picture, a level of hierarchy if you will, into the relationship of the various aspects of our being. In short, it gives us a starting point from which to connect.

As a physiological relationship, going above the head automatically uses the crown chakra as a bridge, thus activating it. In case you get the idea that, it is all a figment of your imagination; the subtle structure of the realms above the head is no less real than the spatial relationship of your organs to one another. A clairvoyant with the necessary awareness, can see this structure above your head as easily as the energy structure within your body.

While this relationship of the realms above the head provides an eternally useful awareness, and is something that can be the means of relating within these realms for many years of practice, keep in mind that there are other ways of accessing these realms. The traditional manner is to access them directly within the chakras of the body. However, this can require decades of practice, along with the transmissions, and even then you may miss the extreme subtlety required, mistaking it for another experience.

Eventually, you will need to gain the direct method of access within the body. You will be able to feel the buddhic realms and their source of spirit from within any chakra in the body. As you continue to open, it is everywhere, the tip of a finger, a point in the air in front of you, a mountain, and a stream— anywhere your awareness activates into that depth. This is the subject of Tantra. The purpose of Eternal Yoga is to introduce you to the direct awareness of these realms of consciousness. Through a few years of cultivating this awareness, you now have the non-dualistic understanding of what you are applying yourself into through the tantric path.

A disadvantage of going above the head is that a mental colorization can easily occur. At first, this mental quality can be put to use.

The mind is fast and can easily expand, which mirrors the buddhic realms very well. You gain an initial experience of an empty feeling more quickly and this gradually helps you to accept emptiness. This kind of emptiness can at times be very uncomfortable, but again, this is put to use on the spiritual path to help us release grasping.

By experiencing the buddhic realms in the same space as the body, this mentalization disappears. You rest in your heart quality more totally.

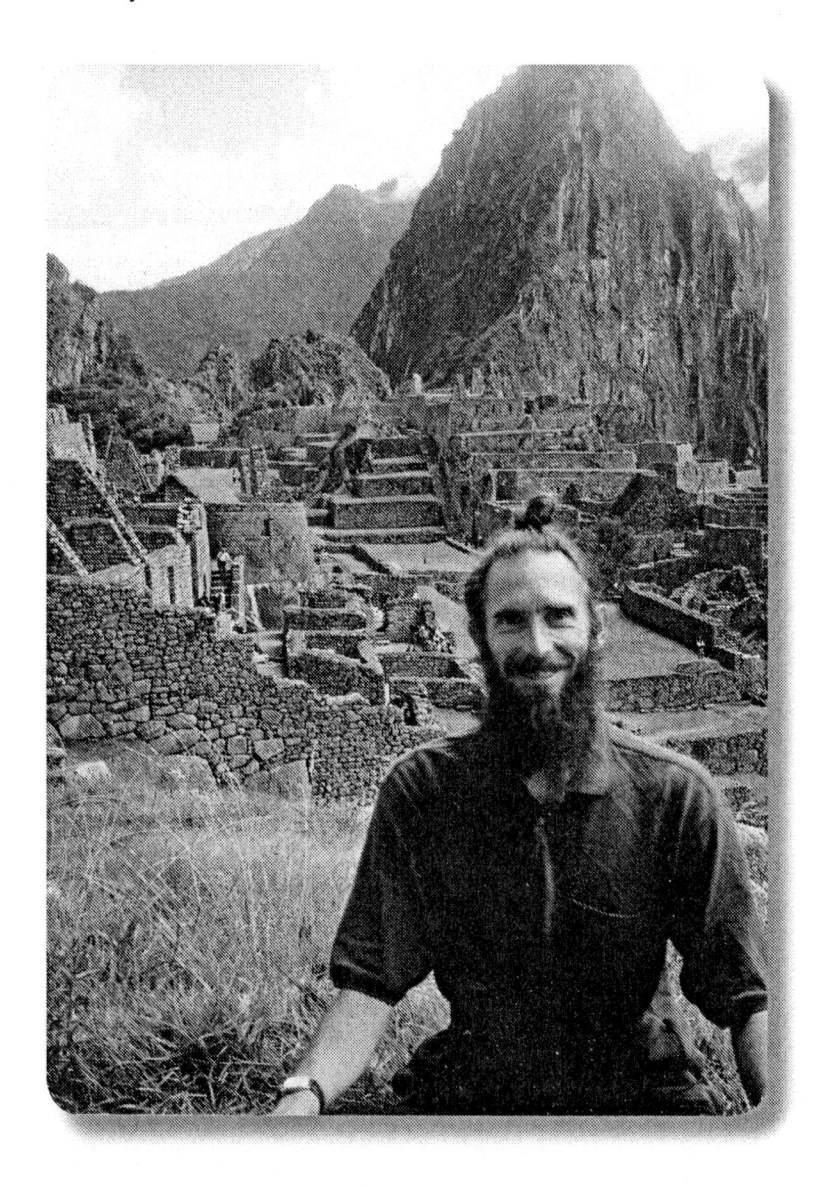

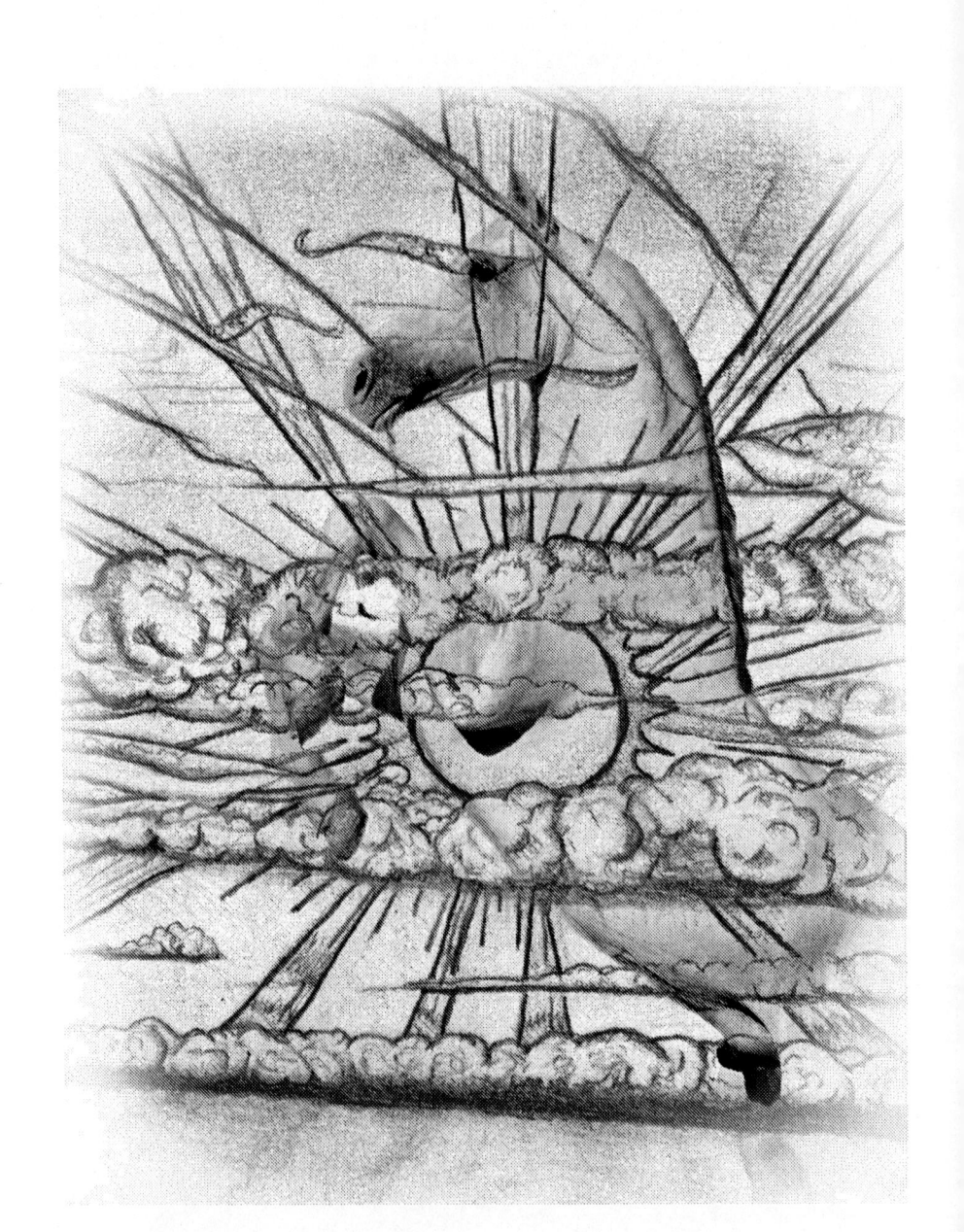

114 Eternal Yoga, Awakening within Buddhic Consciousness

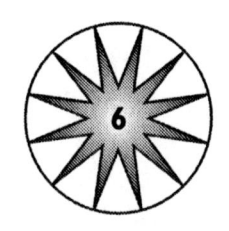

Soul Development through the Rays of Light

Introduction to the Rays

On the tantric path, we receive understanding from the deepest levels of our being and work to integrate this gradually into an outer level of consciousness. Often these depths are so subtle and formless, that it can be difficult to feel the process at all.

To have awareness of our subtlety requires that we are conscious of something. Fortunately, there are ways to bridge this gap, starting with universal qualities such as colors, and characteristics such as strength, determination, and love. If we realize that from our most subtle dimensions to our physical density all is a continuum and thus shares a common ground, then it should be common sense that there will be attributes that are similar within all the various dimensions of our being. The principal difference from one dimension and another is how we perceive. To use the often-quoted example, "A god sees water as nectar, a human as something to drink, and to a hell-being the water is a poisonous substance." Filled with nectar, the god thus experiences life as a flow of nectar, and drinks the nectar. Drinking for nourishment and refreshment, the human for the most part is ignorant of water being anything else. Pain and suffering is the reality of the hell being, so water is also a source of torture. These different perceptions, all of which are valid within their framework, further qualify the underlying quality called water.

Joe, an average human, decides he wants to experience for himself what a god experiences. He has read some fantastic descriptions, but honestly, they are just words. His intention reaches up into his soul, although he is not conscious of it in this way, and while pondering all of this, he notices a glass of water sitting on his bedside table. Oddly, he cannot take his eyes off the glass of water and starts to wonder, "How would a god would see this water."

As he stares at the water, and it being late at night, his mind begins to relax and opens up a bit. His soul is now able to give him a bit of help. Falling asleep, he has a quick, vivid dream of jumping in a pool of water by a mountain stream. It is very refreshing. Energized by the experience, Joe quickly wakes. Only five minutes has passed, yet he feels as if he has slept for hours—so exhilarating.

Everything around has a sparkling quality to it. Instead of running off with his mind, he simply stays with it, and slowly starts to realize, without really thinking about it, heavenly beings, like angels (gods), must experience a lot of bliss. Perhaps to them water is blissful. Connecting together bliss (he is still feeling very energized from the dream) and water creates within him a tangible experience. Joe, our average human, has used water, an everyday universal phenomena, to begin to bridge into another way of perception.

Perhaps of all the sensory stimuli we experience in everyday life, light, being transparent, radiant, and well, light-like, is the easiest to use for the purposes of creating this bridge. To bring further definition, there are many colors of light, and each of these colors can evoke different responses within us. Welcome to the language of the Rays.

The word "ray" has useful connotations. For example, we have the rays of the sun. A ray can be more than just light. It can be warming. There can be qualities, such as strength or penetration. A ray has a certain cosmic association to the word. The language of the rays starts with qualities that we all have experienced. The quality by which we name a ray is like using a pointer. The pointer itself is not the perception we are trying to realize, but it does point us in the right direction.[1] For example, we have the Blue Ray, the Red Ray, and the Green Ray. Each is pointing us in a different direction, that is, they are evoking different qualities within us.

Understanding different rays helps us to round out our spiritual development from different perspectives. As we delve deeper into the qualities of a ray, at times this can seem a bit clumsy, mistaking the name of a ray (its color) for the ray itself. Imagine for a moment, that you lived in a world where cars do not exist. However, in another dimension, there are things that move which mystics call cars and they are all silver in color. The metaphysicians of your world

[1] For the more advanced aspects of Eternal Yoga, it is important to note that we cannot use the rays or visualization of a color to penetrate into the most inner aspect of our spirit. Any type of projection or effort cannot bring us into this consiousness. For this, we need to be in non-dual awareness to find that which we are already. Trying to use the rays or any technique to become non-dual is simply keeping us in a level of separation. Becoming non-dual is simply something that we profoundly become aware of when we are ready to take notice, and thus is something we catch—a transmission.

announce that this ray of cars be named the Silver Ray. Seems to fit, after all, cars, excuse me, moving objects of a strange form, are silver in color. Then lo and behold, in your meditation you see a red car. Hmm, is this not the car ray, why is it red? Red was meant to be the volcano ray. Yet it moves like a car, runs like a car, looks like a car, except it is red. However, in your world red is the name of the ray of volcanoes, not cars.

The essence of that ray was not silver, but cars. Yet in your planet, no one has any concept of a car, so silver is used for the description. Similarly, the essences of the rays are beyond what we have concepts for, i.e., there are no words for it. However, this is a subtle point that does not stop us from starting.

Visualizing a color, noticing the effects, and attuning to the feelings associated with the visualized color are perhaps the best way to introduce oneself to a ray. Blue definitely brings forth a different experience than red. In addition, color is a good way to engage the mind while at the same time deepening it into non-verbal expression.

Depending on how you are connecting with the ray, sometimes it is better to focus on a characteristic other than its color. Which color would you give to the quality of love, compassion, will, penetration...?

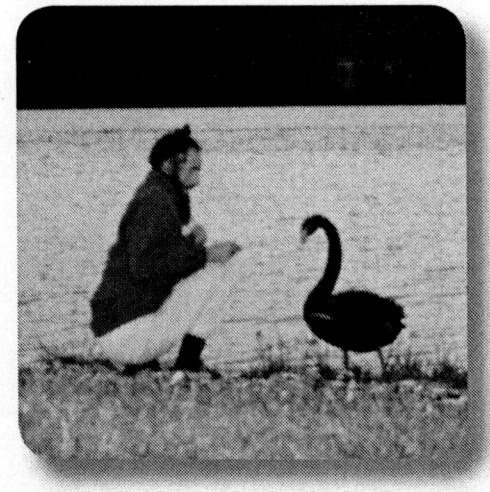

A mature understanding of the rays only comes forth in a sense of wholeness. Within this understanding of wholeness, we can then bring forth greater definition within our various aspects. Each ray is a particular way of expression or mindset, which together makes up our universe as a whole. Where do you draw the boundaries of one ray to the next? When we need distinction to develop definition, each ray can be very different and defined. When we do not need this development, the rays can all be of the same taste. As we refine ourselves into the vastness of consciousness that the Eternal Yoga practices bring, it is important to allow a fluidity of movement between definition and sameness. If we do not allow this fluidity, then we are too stuck in our outer channels, rather than feeling into our depth.[2] The wisdom of how to do this, to be it all, is already contained within the refinement of the space we are moving into through these practices.

We can describe each particular cosmic school of consciousness as a ray of consciousness. We condense all the qualities of the school into a single essence that we can hold in the palm of our hand. The elemental qualities of the universe are each a ray. A simple way to connect, and yet the whole universe is made of these few rays. An example of this is the five buddhic-families referenced within Buddhism.

Earthly and Cosmic Aspects of the Rays, and their Application as a Language of the Soul

Each of the rays has an earthly and cosmic aspect. The earthly aspect is its perception within an everyday context. This is the activity of a ray by the time it has percolated through our subtle nervous system into our tissues, perceptions, thoughts, and emotions.

Within a cosmic ray, there is a heavenly and a transcendent aspect. At times, this difference is obvious. At other times, there is no point in recognizing the difference, because for practical purposes, there is none. An example of the heavenly aspect of a ray would be its experience within the nectars and deep in the chakras. The transcendent cosmic ray is awareness of the ray as it "originates" in buddhic space. This is the true initiation of a ray and the understanding of a ray as an innate quality of the universe.

When I say that the transcendent aspect of a ray is an innate quality of the universe, this does not indicate that you could ever perceive this ray independent of an individualized consciousness embodying it. For example, my initiation into the higher aspects of the Red Ray, was not seeing red, it was seeing Meru in his red aspect

---

[2] We can learn how to see through feeling. Subtle feeling is the direct awareness of our subtly originating pranas of spirit, which many call truth, or knowingness.

appearing within the buddhic realms. Nothing in the universe exists outside of a consciousness either directly embodying it or one that has set it forth in motion. There is no such thing, not a single atom, rock, idea, force, feeling of love, or even space, that exists other than through a consciousness that brought it into being. Not even consciousnesses can exist as an independent entity, a separate quality within the universe. The moment you have consciousness, you have a manifestation, a source of energy. Spirit is pure consciousness, the eternal wellspring of energy and manifestation. When you get into the transcendent aspect of a ray, you are awakening directly to source, where all of this becomes obvious. It is impossible to awaken into spirit, without awakening into the Body of the One, the beings that are awake as spirit. There is no separation at that level. When the appearance of separation occurs, that is when you enter into the illusory perception of the world as existing independently—knock on wood.

When your awareness of a particular ray penetrates into its transcendent cosmic aspect, you will then be able to see through the many requalifications as it supports consciousness down through the layers of awareness. Not only are there gross uses of a ray that result in and from a gross consciousness, there is heavenly ignorance of a ray that usually comes about because of an imbalanced or ignorant perspective from the soul. Conflicts in heaven take place upon the misqualifications of these rays, or aspects of consciousness. Examples of this typically occur in the subtle depths of religious pride, countries, soul groups, and power plays.

The above-mentioned earthly aspect of a ray is not the same as how the ray is used within the earth.[3] Within the earth, a ray can be used in any of its variations, according to its application and who is making the application. For example, the angels typically use the heavenly or cosmic aspects of a ray within the earth, for this is a natural reflection of their refinement.

Within the practice of Eternal Yoga, it is important to awaken to the cosmic aspects of the rays. All the rays have cosmic aspects,

---

[3] There is a chapter in the *Tantra of the Beloved* book on the inner-earth (see appendix).

although some of the rays are seldom grounded into an earthly or terrestrial aspect within the physiology of the human body and subtle energy system. An example of this is the Silver Ray.

For further clarification, think of the rays as aspects of your soul. There are some aspects which find there way into a bodily expression more easily than others. The Red, Orange, and Gold Rays, for example, find there way into a support of the physical body more easily than the Silver Ray. They are characteristics in which the souls of our organs embody upon, with a direct result of being able to digest food, to circulate life-force, to integrate experience, to have sensory organs, etc. Upon these rays we also have an opportunity of further definition, by development of character. In contrast, the rays which remain more in the soul realms, such as the Silver Ray, for the most part have little physiological grounding into the body. The consciousness that they support is just too far beyond what most people can physically, emotionally, and mentally embody upon, although they are understood when we become conscious as a soul.

This is a work in progress, and as we develop within our soul in a continuum with our physical forms, then these more soul-bound rays find a greater expression into the physical, and in the process will greatly transform physical life as we know it.

For your information, there are movements and experiences of cosmic consiousness that are beyond the soul realms and cannot be given an association with a color or defined by a characteristic. These are experientially embodied within the light beyond the light, beyond the soul, in what we call the Body of the One. As a prelude, how would you describe the radiant field of emptiness (sunyata), the oneness, in terms of a soul ray? What about primordial space—the creation of souls who are never born nor ever die—holding Spirit in the palm of your hand—the Oneness of all there is, in infinite fields of multiplicity? None of this is a static consciousness, rather a reality-movement-radiance-effect that is indescribable by a soul not blissfully awakened far beyond itself and definitely not within the conventional notion of time and space by a physically bound personality. In the framework of the One, all things are possible, and do occur.

Coming back to Terra firma, or at least to the fields of Soul-delight, a ray may look entirely different depending on the level of awareness in which you focus within it. For example, you may have a different experience of the Gold Ray when you meditate upon it through your solar plexus, versus at the top of your head. The language of the rays is not unlike the Taoist use of Yin and Yang. Yin and Yang by themselves are only useful in a relative understanding, and what is yin and yang changes according to the particular use. As another example, consider acupuncture. When an acupuncturist refers to liver energy, they are not necessarily referring to the liver itself, rather a kind of energy in the body most associated with the liver. You can have your spleen organ removed and live, but if you remove your spleen energy, then you will die.

The rays are useful to understand ourselves from a place of light and transparency, which is the reason that when we refer to the rays we mostly do so by color. When we talk of elemental qualities from the perspective of the rays, we are talking about these elemental qualities from a place of light and consciousness. Even when we are talking about the earthly qualities of a ray, we are still doing so from a place of energy and light. If we say that we experience Green Tara or White Tara, we are talking about the spirit of Tara on the Green Ray, or the spirit of Tara as a white quality. Because we connect with the rays, they are a natural language to use within the Eternal Yoga practices. The rays as spirit are an active principle, not a passive side effect. When we say Green Tara, we are not talking about a splotch of green paint, rather a profound Being communicating through an incredibly alive medium, which is not separate from her. If we are focusing on developing the Gold Ray in our solar plexus, we are not talking about a passive principle. It will do little good simply to put some gold paint on your stomach and forget about it. Rather we are saying, feel, visualize, and experience yourself as gold within your solar plexus. What is the effect? What happens if we feel golden pranas of the earth gather there?

If you try to understand the rays solely by reading, studying, studying, studying and analyzing, you will get nothing of any spiritual value. This is an experiential language, slowly matured through practice and life experience. It is an applied language, i.e., you visualize blue and see what happens. We cannot understand blue by reading the word blue—it is only be seeing blue. When we see blue, in various contexts, we develop various associations through our response to this vision. By the power of association, we emotionally bridge the gaps, and eventually we are clear enough to perceive directly the nature of existence. You enter into a deep space within yourself and start bringing forth a fabric of the rays in order to awaken more fully. It is not that we need to have our experience match another's experience; rather it is bridging the gap from unconsciousness into consciousness, by which the concept of the rays serve us. It is the application itself that is important, not the validity of one definition over another.

By understanding the rays as modes of consciousness operating through the continuum of existence, we can clear up a lot of confusion. For example, many people connect to the Blue Ray through association of its transcendent aspect. This is a refined mental quality of connected thought and space. However, you may also connect with the Blue Ray as a watery strength such as grounded within the kidneys, or a spacious aspect such as in the heart or throat. Each of the rays also has a cosmic aspect that originates from within the buddhic body. Mastery within the cosmic aspects of the rays does not come forth until a person is fluent within those realms and free of gross distortions that would force a limited perspective. Otherwise, they will be qualified in a lesser light. Some of the rays are only available from the cosmic levels. That is, eating more food, studying about something, or going for a walk is not going to generate awareness of these rays within your being.

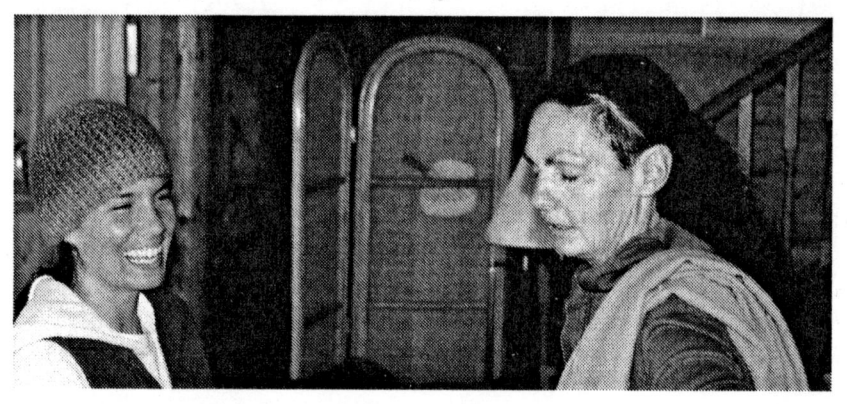

The rays crystallize into a language of the soul through familiarity with them. The best way to become familiar with a ray is to meditate with it. Thus, visualize its color within and around you. Wear some clothes of that color. Sense and feel it. What animals, beings, Masters, or qualities do you sense? What are your dreams like? Are there particular places in your body you gravitate to when visualizing a color? What are your emotions like? This growing awareness should be cultivated over time to gain greater maturity and fluidity within the ray. By meditating on the radiant purity of a ray, you purify that aspect of your self.

The beauty of the rays is when you become somewhat fluent in all of them; they are all experienced as aspects of your presence. In this way, you heal personality splits and enjoy a greater sense of wholeness.

A Prelude to the Descriptions of the Rays

In many of the descriptions of the rays that follow, various teachings are included, that at first may not appear to be overly connected with the ray. For example, a visualization may be given that would seem equally valid using another color, or a teaching on the Devas may be included.

This is in accordance with how teachings actually unfold with continued focus within a ray. Each of these rays is also the essence of a school, and as such, there are various teachings emphasized within each of the schools.

In addition to the positive gifts of each ray, also addressed are the shortcomings that may occur through a ray becoming overly dominant, through ignorance, or through misuse of the ray itself. As the rays are a language by which we can round out our soul development, it is important that we are able to recognize not only the strengths of our soul, but also its deficiencies, if we are truly to grow into a fullness of light.

Within the tantric mandala of the Ascended Masters in service to our planet, there are particular Masters who are well known for their overseeing of soul development in the rays. Each of these Masters are well versed in the use of all the rays; however, their specialized service within one or two rays is a combination of long experience within those teachings. This continues as an ongoing service to their students within that teaching.

Many of the Masters within this mandala are emanations of archangels who hold a particular quality in the universe. This mandala has been at work for a very long time, creating the inner etheric structure of the earth, resulting in how this Earth serves us all. In this creation, various Masters take responsibility for particular aspects, reflective of their own essence. The Masters effortlessly work as and through each other, as this is a quality of the Body of the One.

The book, Tantra of the Beloved (see appendix) describes these and other Masters in more depth. Also, look at our web site, www.sacredmountainretreat.org for pictures and recent articles on the Masters.

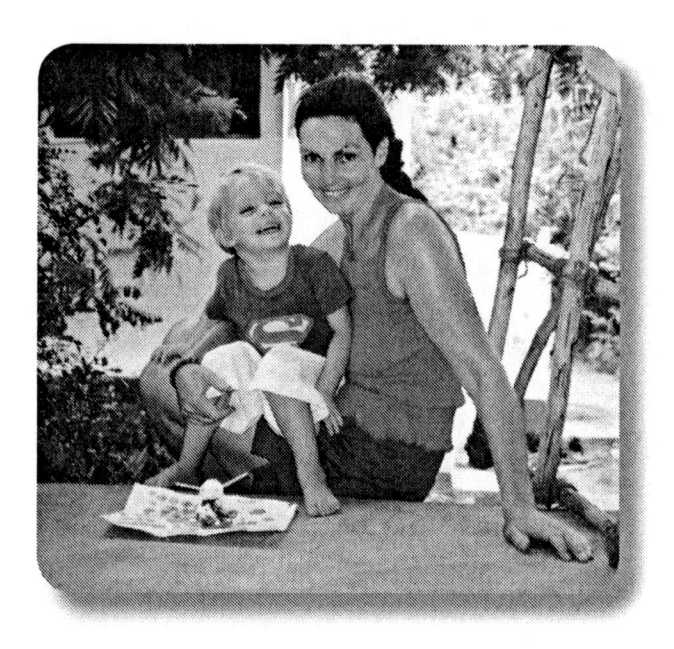

Blue

The Blue Ray, in its cosmic aspect, is an essence of mind originating as awareness of primal space. With a developed Blue Ray, within your mind, it is easy to move through time and space. There is a quick intelligence with an innate ability to understand how a thought relates to other thoughts and scenarios, including the underlying space of the thought itself. This results in extreme sensitivity, although not necessarily of a high-strung nature.

Taken down a notch, the blue flame becomes etheric space surrounding and permeating ideas and forms. This is the blue light often seen through the third eye. As such, it carries the dynamic blueprint of which the various terrestrial rays bring forth manifestation.

Having access to the larger vision, it carries a sense of transcendence and a purity that only comes from beyond the personality. A person emanating the full command of this ray, while remaining true to its function in the Oneness, is a natural leader.

Those who have long served on the Blue Ray greatly value loyalty, clarity and integrity. There is a deep peace in the Blue Ray as it helps us beyond limited personality. Bodhisattva ideals and service to the greater good are second nature within those of a predominant Blue Ray disposition. The bigger picture is always prevalent.

The Blue Ray is close to cosmic consciousness, such as the silver and cosmic-white rays. There is a natural connection within the fluidity of the water element. While not an absolute, there is a natural affinity of a Blue Ray personality with the bright and tantric aspect of the Orange Ray.

When the Blue Ray becomes too predominant, then we can easily become too aloof or idealistic. Emotional integration is lacking and righteousness starts dictating our life. Sacrificing the little things for the bigger picture all the time does not let the perfection play its part.

Blue is often associated with mind essence, which is a subtle ability to notice and qualify existence from beyond a level of intellectuality. Some practices color the essence flame within the heart as blue, denoting the mind at rest in its primordial quality. The mental power of this ray, in its maturity, does not create a stifling domination. You exhibit a working balance in everything you do. The crystal-clear mind is quick, very, very quick, yet instigates nothing out of Divine timing, for it is sensitive and complete in itself. By anchoring the mind in Divine Presence, nothing can compel it into conflict, separation, or deceit.

Blue is transcendent, unattached, cooling, purifying, divine, peaceful, exacting, aware, connected, patient, precise, meditative and when its introvert nature is overcome by a full embrace of life, it empowers leadership and excellence. In its highest truth, it is of the light beyond the light, denoting pure self-awareness.

The blue light brings forth the truth in any situation. In its purity, it is unshakeable. Connected with the underlying matrix of thoughts and energies that form inner space and time, there is an ability to influence how one thought associates with another. So blue, in a sense, forms the ethers of itself. The sensitivity of the Blue Ray is a natural protection, because you are aware of what is occurring and can take action on a very deep level, orchestrating the ethers in cooperation to the best course of action. In this sensitivity, your thoughts will be able to radiate along the best routes of association.

The Blue Ray, while able to hold an essence understanding, needs the clothing of other energies, other rays, to become visible and manifest. Often a Blue Ray personality holds the possibility, experiencing little in terms of outer phenomena, while others who are more conversant in the terrestrial-rays have many visions and experiences. Of course, as a predominant Blue Ray person brings forth these other qualities within him or her self, they will then clothe this light for themselves.

Blue is an inner color and brings forth a meditative atmosphere. Its integrity can bring great strength and its purity keeps the will on track. It is a ray of precision and exactness. The ability to sense the route of association of one thought or energy to another allows you to penetrate. This gives you the consciousness to facilitate greater subtle alignment, holding the positive energetic and selfless support necessary to bring forth greater unity and understanding.

Blue is a color of loyalty, by the right of commitment. Precision, rhythmic movements and breath patterns bring out a blue energy in the body's magnetic field. Such exercise strengthens the body and the nervous system. Blue is a color of expanse, such as the sky and the ocean. It indicates spiritual development beyond the pull of the emotions and thus has great patience.

Being on track with spiritual purpose and the constant reflection of inner purity, such as, "May the best happen for all beings," creates and holds a strong blue energy. Being able to hold it all is a quality of the blue expression. The blue command is no-nonsense, to the point, exact and precise, self-empowered and transcendent of all belittlement, it radiates a loving equilibrium and fluidity. Because it makes its decisions from a deep level beyond personality, it can outwardly appear as ruthless.

Deepening the Blue Ray is a meditative affair, reflecting the purity upon which you connect with your sense of divinity. Speaking your highest truth is equally important, lest your truth never incarnate. Overcoming doubt and being able to feel with purity is the only way of sustaining this development—I AM.

Those who are predominant in the Blue Ray through many lifetimes and have a devic personality, often have to overcome doubt, and once they do, are far beyond it. This is because the penetration and insight so easily obtained brings a deep knowingness. This knowingness, originating from beyond a level of common vision, is often a kind of very deep feeling. Yet, until there is enough filling out on the other rays, there is not enough development to support bringing forth this knowingness, particularly in regards to its impact upon all the invested emotional energies of the world. [4]

While a Blue Ray person must often speak out and communicate to fulfill their soul purpose, the sound of the Blue Ray itself is silence. This is the touchstone, upon which you can access your balance and connectivity on this ray. Without this inner eloquence of silence, then you are not actually in the depths of the Blue Ray, even if you think of yourself as otherwise.

---

[4] This development includes emotional clarity and strength, along with perceiving the perspective of each ray within the essence of its truth, so that it comes forth in an integrated manner that is of benefit. The overcoming of doubt in this scenario is not a doubt of what one knows, rather, doubt as to the fullness of its truth, which includes its ability to benefit people, while retaining its essence to cut through any delusions. There is sometimes a practical emotional strengthening required as well, in order to have the supportive force necessary to stand behind this truth, when there are those who would rather you did not. This is a well known topic within the blue ray school.

It is imperative that a person with an active mind, fueled by Blue Ray tendencies, practice vigorous exercise, such as dynamic yoga, skilled application of the breath, long, deep meditation and lives a meaningful life. Otherwise, the mental stimulation has nowhere to express itself properly. Thus, imbalance, distortion, headiness and disempowerment are the result, all of which undermine the potential within this ray.

The Blue Ray clarity is not initially one of vision (this comes later); it is a deeper attunement that of all the senses, feeling is the closest to it (seeing through feeling). It has a formless depth. Without consciously remaining in this depth, the exactness of the Blue Ray personality, through its acute perception, can create an overly analytical, sharp, and critical disposition. This limited mindset interferes with your ability to feel, and thus experience clarity. Because of the giving nature of the Blue Ray (always the bigger picture), there are often deep emotional issues resulting from our own personal needs being ignored. Of course, this can lead to resentment, emotional pain through constant misunderstanding by others, disconnection, and overcompensation through wanting our needs to be met by others liking us. As this healing occurs, the mind through feeling finds its resting place in the heart; thus, awareness expands to the wholeness of your being in all its divine and apparently mundane aspects.

When there is enough Self-Love and healing, the mind expands beyond the need for the outer self to control everything around it. Thus, you surrender into your wholeness and become the commanding presence at one with all the rays.

When the mind ignites in your cosmic heart, it brings a joy-filled presence of the indescribable beauty and perfection of the universe, at One with all your higher mental faculties of discernment, connectivity and knowingness.

Developing your Blue Ray enhances higher mental awareness, projection and communication. The strong, incorruptible, penetrating rod of this ray from above into your physical awareness anchors an angelic grounding of subtle activity. Begin by attuning to the Blue Ray in the throat or the third eye. The blue flame colors the subtle energy residing deep within the spinal chord. As a transcendent and advanced manifestation, blue can become the color of every chakra and channel.

A person favoring the Blue Ray will naturally look to yogic exercise, breathing, etc., with a feeling sensitivity to energy in relation to the body. Energy awareness is the key this type of person will use throughout the yogic process. Typically, a Blue Ray personality without development on the other rays, through their sensitivity, will often hold a psychic space for others, yet lack the inner vision to see content within that energy field.

So far, a deep, radiant, royal blue has been our focus. The various shades of blue have vastly different properties depending on the context of their application and perception. For example, a soft mid-blue, a mixture of white and blue, is used in very subtle devic kingdoms and when awakened in the thymus, genitals, and within the channels is indescribable and of an incredibly high level of advancement. Yet this color of blue, when it has a washed-out dull feeling to it, often results from a lack of commitment and definition. Therefore, it is the energy of the ray, not just its visual color, which is important.

The Ascended Master El Morya is often looked upon as a role model for the Blue Ray, helping to oversee those who excel upon it. El Morya has also been known as King Arthur, a medicine women in the black hills of South Dakota, Apollo, Guru Gobind Singh of the Sikhs, Rishi Dush Dhaman of Hemkunt Sahib, and Vairochana of Tibet. He obtained his full ascension as Guru Gobind Singh, although often uses a taller turbaned image as El Morya. His Twin Ray, also very accomplished on the Blue Ray, is Yeshe Tsogyel.

El Morya and Yeshe Tsogyel oversee the crystal grid within the planet. They are supreme protectors and have trained many yogic warriors. The famed 40 liberated ones under Guru Gobind Singh serve under El Morya in a very active manner for this function, as do many under Yeshe Tsogyel. The beauty of the orchestration of these Masters in action is a privilege to behold.

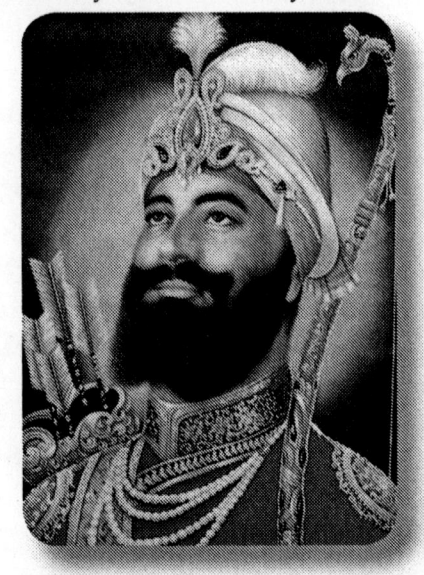

Decrees

"I AM the purity commanding forth every cell of creation into the Perfection—I AM."

"I AM the alignment of cosmic truth into the outer thoughts, activity and feelings."

"I AM the transcendence of all belittlement, the Love which is infinitely patient, the Sight to see and the Wisdom which never flinches."

"I AM the penetration and the anchoring of truth brought forth as my Presence, which remains regardless of what comes and goes."

"I AM the activation of my higher mental body and its Radiant Presence grounded into my physical awareness."

Gold

The Gold Ray is the higher-mind creating prana. The prana of the Gold Ray transforms us into the action and energy of divine fulfillment. This gives a natural confidence, bringing forth the kingdom of the will. Within its own domain, this preference for action honors or tolerates patience only when it is perceived to serve greater action.

In its highest personification, the Gold Ray is the very idea of radiance itself. A Gold Ray person is confident in the use of emotion as an expression of movement. The Gold Ray opens a further support for telepathic qualities. It is quite common for people with development on the Gold Ray to have a natural rapport with animals. These qualities are not unique to the gold ray; however, this ray enhances these qualities in a special way. Because of its radiant, giving, and earthy quality, a Gold Ray person often has a big heart.

Gold brings clarity from the higher-mind and strength in the etheric body. This is equal to a great "keep up." It helps to give substance to the vast divinity of blue, as both work in close communion with the will of the One. It works with the radiance of purple in royalty. With green it is very healing. With white it is initiating and bright. It gives direction to red. The gold, orange and Red Rays can easily co-mingle within their functions.

Krishna is often painted in gold, blue and black. This is symbolic of the tantric dance of the fusion channel, gold being prana, blue the cosmic template and black signifying the formless origin able to work beyond limitations of a particular personality. It is the Love Dance becoming the masculine and feminine reality, yet remaining non-dual in nature. It embraces all levels of apparent duality by enjoying the dance.

It has been said that the element of gold is no less than the frozen rays of the sun. Actually, all the elements contain the frozen rays of the sun; however, in gold they are in great abundance. This is the solar energy found within the ninth realm above the head.

Overly emphasizing the Gold Ray so that development of the other rays suffer, results in blind-ambition, over-confidence, lack of humility and disregard for the values of purity and integrity. In short, one thinks of oneself as a law unto oneself and this blinds us to further progress.

A willful, determined, confident personality who always ends up learning life's lessons the hard way, demonstrates the Gold Ray out of balance. The individual will is out of alignment with spirit, creating a self-perpetuating spiritual blindness. The victory of life is to remain in radiant awareness of Oneness, of your source constantly bringing forth beauty, fullness, and perfection—never feeling or allowing the outer personality as a law unto itself.

Inner growth includes all the rays within the Great Presence. There is only enlightened will and distorted will. Enlightened will is the Divine movement of the universe. Distorted will is karmic activity of a person who, in that moment, has not yet found the Oneness. It is all a matter of purely held alignment with the God-self.

In this unity, you become the manifest glory of your divinity. Consciously hold the outer in check by choosing unity over disunity, alignment over dominance, purity over covert tendencies. The moment that you become aware of a split between the outer and the inner, your duty is self-correction.

I am not talking about unity of social consciousness, an alignment with untruth, or a puritanical morality. When obstructions, such as these, actively try to block the higher unity and higher movement, we need courage to overcome them. Unfortunately, much confusion results from trying to sort out what is what. While a judgmental energy holds us back through our own limitation, so can a misguided fear of appearing judgmental. There are those who move in a distorted and destructive way, and say, "Do not judge me," as a way of disarming those who might try to stop them from their pollution of the world. The highest light is the fabric that everything in creation rests upon. Align your knowingness within that light and shine it through your presence into all the corners of the world. You have already won when there is nowhere else to go. Distortions will bring their own downfall, as there is no alignment with the underlying support. The solution is our own inner growth, our own unity. Keep moving forward with an open heart of a warrior, and release any unnecessary pride in the process.

Please, do not become confused with disempowered statements such as, "I know nothing, spirit does it all," or with being an unconscious trance channel. These serious splits need healing. Penetrating into your presence flame within the depths and source of your body-temple is what brings forth unity and self-radiant consciousness.[5] Our egoic separation is what prevents us from knowing God. In the Ascended state, our limited personality dies. You can never achieve this through trying to get rid of your personality, such as through the idea of renunciation or denial. Rather, it is active absorption through love and surrender into our depths, into the Body of the One. It is becoming more, not less. It is a penetration. You evolve into the readiness of it. In this way, we become transparent and aware of this light, and become it. Then what was previously our ego, becomes an expression of divine-light, in the only way it ever can, through an individual such as you. However, the whole concept of individuality changes—you can experience the Masters within you

---

[5] Self-radiant consciousness is primal to its qualifications. Everyday consciousness is constantly qualified by the world in which you live. For example, if you are tired, you may not feel as clear and crisp as after a good night's sleep. What you eat, see, taste, etc., constantly qualifies how consciously aware you are. There is, however, a state of consciousness that is primal to all this, and that is simply the awareness of being conscious. Regardless of how you outwardly feel, you can train yourself to become aware that you are a self-conscious being. This awareness has a subtle continuity of radiance that underlies everything else. Having this freedom, you can learn to remain awake in this state and then explore any area that you fancy, beyond the confines of the outer limitations imposed on conscious awareness.

and as you. You must refine yourself enough so that your true light can work as you. Only you can initiate this alignment. It is God, who is always awake, awakening to itself. In that victory you can never be corrupted and there is always marvel and gratitude in the spontaneous creative outpouring of your joy-filled Divine Essence, I AM.

To correct self-blinding misuse of will on the gold ray, you must first see and correct any basic distortions of the Red and Green Rays. The Red Ray distortions include grabbing and misplacement of power. Green Ray distortions include jealousy, covert activity through subtle manipulation, abuse of the feminine nature, and irreverence of timing despite claims otherwise. These types of distortion compel a distorted use of will and pranic force.

Releasing the feeling of struggle opens the heart to a world that includes and is beyond the outer senses. The inner eloquence of Perfection blossoms forth—you become it by being it. This eloquence takes into consideration more than a contracted, selfish view ever will, thus it needs your depth and trust to see its wisdom.

You can apply the Gold Ray just as easily for earthly pranas or for heavenly outpourings, and thus it is a natural vehicle of integrating earth and heaven.

The Gold Ray is commonly developed through the solar plexus, navel, heart and various chakras in the head. Many chi-kung exercises are good for developing the gold ray, if consciously used in this way, as is a deep connection with the pranas of the earth. The Gold Ray in the body helps us to be strong and confident. In its cosmic aspects, it can form an eye of seeing and a manifestation of very tangible prana from pure consciousness.

The Gold Ray characterizes radiant determination and an optimistic attitude with the energy to match that determination. If you source the confidence of the Gold Ray from the outer personality, rather than spirit, then it becomes a yellow color. This is the intellect manipulating the body's prana, as if it was creating it. It is not the true effortless radiance of the higher centers. The intellect in this way gives a false strength, which eventually weakens the body and mind through hardship and misunderstanding.

As you reach a fuller expression through the top of your head, through trust in your spirit, a richer, golden quality strengthens the entire body with its radiance, willingness and Divine Love. Gold is a strong component of the higher mental radiance, exuding an eternal youthfulness with a cheerful, playful quality, giving confidence and energy for activity. The gold light can bring forth wonderful awareness of the ninth realm above the head.

The "rays of the sun" are the nuclear forces within an atom. While physicists discover in these forces particular qualities necessary for the stability of our physical creation, the essence of these forces can also act in intelligent ways, through the embodiment of a Master, that are outside theorized law.

Without willingness, there is no application. Without application, there is no experience. Without experience, there is no realization. Without realization, there is a continuation of unconscious thought and behavior.

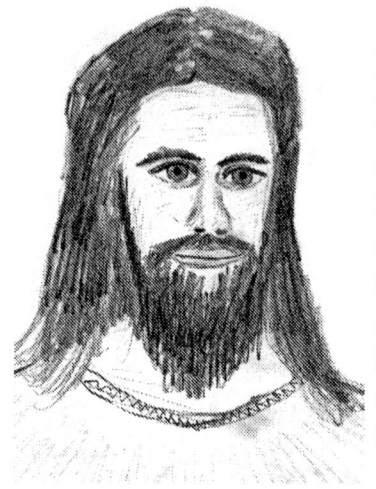

There are many distinguished Gold Ray Masters. The Ascended Master Koothumi is often looked upon as the principle overseer of the Gold Ray for this planet. Koothumi has also been Saint Francis of Assisi, Guru Ram Dass of the Sikhs, a significant player in the development of Tibetan Buddhism, and Moses. He has a very deep laugh. His Twin Ray is Saint Claire. Jesus is also known for his strong Gold Ray development.

Decrees

"I AM the Way, the Truth and the Light."

"I AM growing stronger daily in my I AM Presence."

"I AM the Ever-Expanding Perfection."

"I AM the confidence, radiance and strength of my infinite being."

Red

The Red Ray brings forth strength and definition. It creates a no-nonsense, practical and vital disposition, capable of dealing with everything from the little things in life to leading a revolution.

By visualizing this ray within the body, it becomes more responsive and transparent on a cellular level. As a source of energy, red can be used to energize and to consume, such as by fire. Use of the Red Ray naturally activates the right side of the body, making you more outgoing, able to continue through life's challenges, and to excel.

A deep application of the Red Ray has within it both masculine and feminine qualities. By combining the Red and White rays together, you will enhance the effect of strength, as red helps to activate the nectar quality of the White Ray.

When the Red Ray become too dominant, which for a personality driven by it, is easy to do, it results in insensitivity and a forward drive that becomes obsessive, such as power-mad. A mature soul can purposefully use this quality to blast through obstacles; however, most of us will end up making more obstacles than we started with.

The Red Ray brings definition in the physical and thus it will naturally stimulate interest in food, sex, physical fitness, monetary power and physical presence. A great mistake is feeling that the physical world is the source of your strength and existence. From such a distorted perspective, you give the physical world a power that it does not possess. Governing your world in such a way is like finding your way in a dimly lit room with only partial vision. The false sense of power or dominion over a world limited to, "If I don't see it, it ain't real," can bring a person to the mistaken strategy of becoming a law unto themselves.

Knowing your deeper existence brings recognition of the command that your higher Presence has over every aspect of your physical and subtle existence. It is only by sincerely identifying with your deeper essence, in a continuous fashion, that you physically gain the commanding and harmonizing power to direct your sensory and willful desires. In this integration you also gain wisdom as to your emotional fulfillment.

It is the challenge and responsibility of every individual to define themselves from the presence and purity of their own light.

The highest use of the Red Ray is in service. Its non-mental approach makes it a natural for devotion and when put to use, can accomplish great benefits. When this ray can be of service to the higher workings, then it is in correct balance.

While red, like any of the rays, can be visualized anywhere in the body, particularly good places to start with are your root center, navel area, heart, throat, and at times as a red flame in the third eye. You can also illumine the entire inside of the body with red, which creates an intimacy and helps you to see. This is particularly good for those who avoid definition. An advanced application is its use in activating the nectars, as we go deeper into our subtle existence. As such, the ray is applied principally within the central channel and various channels in the body.

Some spiritual traditions avoid use of the Red Ray altogether, even going so far as classifying it as some kind of lower evolution, or dark quality, not to be used. This is total nonsense, for you only have to witness some of the greatest of the Ascended Masters in their use of this ray to realize otherwise.

Often this approach originates because of the presentation of a high teaching when the students are simply not developed enough to bring that teaching into a full integration with their life, not only on a personal level, but in regards to society as a whole. Bringing in the Red Ray lights up many areas, including our passions, sex, ambition, and the body in general. In the course of the teaching, a decision is made that it is easier to simply leave out that whole side. Over the years, a pattern is set, and continues forth into a religious or organizational structure, which of course disempowers it in the long run.

There is some wisdom in the above approach, it is wise not to overly emphasize the Red Ray until a maturity has been gained in the higher centers. While red has long been associated with the tantric path, this association is over-stressed. Prematurely stimulating too much sexual or passionate energy, and seeking their resolution, is not the tantric path, but simply a play of the senses and juices, with no long-term spiritual benefit.

When you are ready, the true initiation into the Red Ray comes from the buddhic realms, not from the base centers. When you understand the Red Ray from this level, then you can cut through misunderstanding upon it much more quickly, and direct the increased vitality towards a more fulfilling result—spiritual liberation. Red is not just a body-orientated quality, it is used in realms far beyond the body as well.

A spiritually dull Red Ray personality can have a, "The physical is all there is," attitude, along with the insensitivity that comes with that attitude. As you awake on the Red Ray, this insensitivity disappears and, while you remain present in the physical, you become much more transparent and responsive. In this transparency, you are automatically aware that there is more than just yourself, and that there is a subtle dimension at work.

In the beginning of your practice with the Red Ray, give it some notice, but do not overdo it. As you develop in meditative awareness, visualize the Red Ray originating from above the head as a radiant image of yourself. Let it pour into the body, every cell of it, spiritualizing the body. This practice will give you all the benefits of the Red Ray, yet keep it under the governorship of your higher self. You will still have to go through all the cleansing, look at all the images, accept and embrace all your passions, everything—with the important addition that there is no split from the upper centers, which will guide you in greater harmony.

An effort to develop the Red Ray before your penetration into transcendent consciousness is not much different from countless lifetimes of building a worldly kingdom in ignorance of the higher union.

Establishing a new model of Red Ray activity, based on purity and incorporating the Red Ray anchored from budhic awareness is one of the most important agendas in bringing forth the cleansing and elevation of life on Earth. Clearing misuse of the Red Ray, particularly in the dharmas, religions, and some of their charismatic leaders, is an important task at hand today—that purity may dictate the best course of each individual. While a sincere desire to grow and develop on all the rays goes a long way in keeping use of the Red Ray in check, it involves a lot of subtle penetration to clear the root issues necessary for the karma-free grounding of this ray. As you come forth on this ray without guidance from your higher Presence, it is easy to quickly become actively or passively entangled in the thick web of collective Red Ray karmas on this planet.

The healthy function of the Red Ray is in service to the Higher Plan. This often includes a natural inclination towards devotion and worship. When the Red Ray personality becomes egotistically centered, it begins to push and use its strength towards getting what it wants, while remaining blind to the higher wisdom. For this higher wisdom, the Red Ray must look to the Blue Ray template and Green Ray timing for its guidance.

The fusion of the Red Ray in service and alignment to the Green Ray results in a maroon color, like that worn by Tibetan monks. To the gold light it combines as an act of beauty. To the violet light it recognizes itself already combined with the Blue Ray and hails the eloquence and wisdom of this ray. Softened by the universal prana of the white light hails the color of pink.

While there are many outwardly-known teachers using the Red Ray to create dominance and charisma, few have shown its actual mastery from a higher viewpoint. Examples of Ascended Masters who have helped bring forth a purification of the Red Ray upon the planet through their embrace of it include Ramakrishna (a very great tantric adept), Meru (also known as Rama), and VajraYogini.

Another area of distortion prevalent in the Red Ray is in the work ethic. While a healthy ability to apply yourself towards constructive activity is a great strength, the use of work as a one-sided approach to life has held more than one soul in the bondage of struggle. The presence of struggle is not a sign of spiritual understanding, rather it is the activity of the ego trying to assert itself, resisting movement, or creating a niche for itself out of alignment with your greater purpose.

Many people must embrace this healing and find the soul-driven activity that nourishes them and others on every level. Its test is simple. Do you find excitement in what you are doing, does it serve some deeper purpose for you? It means letting go of a limited way of being by redefining service as Awakened Love and work as your active application for upliftment, joy, and excitement of Divine purpose. True service never was and never will be the activity wherein a person supports or perpetuates the limitations of social-consciousness.

Finding your God-Presence brings great joy and purpose to whatever you do, through the sheer quality of just being that Essence. Work implies a discipline to support or improve life that at times, means you do it anyway, even if it is not in your joy to do so. This gives grit and the ability to apply yourself, to keep up, and the development of self-worth and esteem.

Regular avenues of karmic-participatory work can serve you and others for awhile, but at some point on the spiritual path you gain a greater freedom. The way that you see this world, its karmas and the true source of its support, means that you no longer need place yourself in areas of work that have little spiritual depth or meaning to them. You have become free of these levels of karmic interaction and part of gaining this freedom is to break free of the Red Ray distortions around the concept of work.

The Earth is eventually to become your Ascension-ground. This is true for all souls who have committed to the collective Light within Her. First, however, you must free yourself from the Earth as a karma-ground by becoming free of karmic participation.

Karmic participation is when you bind yourself to limited activities and relationships which you know are not of your highest light. Yet you continue, because you do not feel, trust, or know that you can create your life in a better way. You continue because you have not yet healed yourself within a certain limited arena. In healing and giving yourself permission to express your higher purpose, the Earth becomes a kind of playground. Finally, as you gain the inner victory, it becomes the place of applying that victory to its full outer manifestation—your Ascension-ground.

Trust in your light that you will be supported in doing what is right for you. There is a limited viewpoint which condemns those who do not follow its brand of work ethic as "lazy." To a spiritually motivated person, the word "lazy" does not even exist. Yet there can be periods in your life when the current is running very deep and the attention is not so focused on outer things. To a person not yet awakened and skilled enough inside to follow this current through the inner spaces, that might mean a lot of time lying around integrating and getting in touch with what is going on. This is an important time when consciously respected and applied. It is advised not to let it slip into lethargy.

My beloved and I have a saying at times, "The less we do, the more that gets done." What needs to be understood is that in this condition, the inner work and penetration is occuring to such a great degree that diluting it through outer distraction lessens what is accomplished through it. We also say "There is no rest for the conscious." In truth, "I AM that which never sleeps."

A lazy person is one who is not able to change, who sabotages their own success, and wants to keep things just the way they are. A lazy person does not want to see what is blocking them, to feel what is holding them back, or to make the effort to change. In fact, some people work very hard at being lazy, even working several full-time jobs at once rather than looking within through their creative power and applying a strength of self-belief to create change in the real and often hidden issues of their life. Dedication to an outer cause of work can become a smokescreen to prevent looking at deep emotional issues; there will always seem to be reasons of social consciousness that it must be this way. The message is: first the inner work and clarity, then the outer activity. Neither a lazy person nor a person driven and obsessed by work have the time to find the way of balance. (I do not intend to "put down" those who genuinely find great purpose and reason, in physically and spiritually working long days and nights. Such souls are often right on track. I often do this, as required. This is something that must be genuinely known as perfect for that time.)

The Red Ray quickens, purifies, and strengthens the physical and astral bodies, helping bring forth definition. The Red Ray also is very good at dissolving dross. The dual nature of the Red Ray, to strengthen or to dissolve, is accomplished by how it is used and the feeling with which it is qualified. For example, a red energy active in the body can bring muscular strength, or it can bring a great cleansing resulting in a temporary feeling of weakness. The qualitative effects that the Red Ray has on your body also depends on the being from which the ray is sourced from. Do you feel your own presence behind it, or someone else, a role model, or perhaps an opponent? You also qualify the Red Ray by how comfortable you feel with using it.

Red denotes power, physical vitality and health. It helps in physical discipline and labor, bringing cheerfulness. It can purify the physical and emotional bodies through its vibrant visualization. Meditating with the color red stimulates the astral (emotional) dimension and quickens the movement of energy in the body, giving it a tangible feeling. It helps to have the red light in the body to give it the strength to sit for long periods of time.

A bright red light may be used to clear obstructions in the subtle energy channels. Used in this way, it gives the ability to "see" inside your physical body and feel its energy.

The strength and power aspect of the Red Ray helps people who work physically for a living, as well as those who work with responsibility upon the Earth plane. It enhances physical health, charisma and connectivity, particularly when in service to a spiritually refined existence.

A strong Red Ray person is fully present and has no hesitation in drawing upon all the support given in the physical plane to support that presence. Those who think they are above it all, disempower themselves through lack of connectivity. Before the Red Ray can be strong, a person must make a spiritual decision that they really want to be here on planet earth!

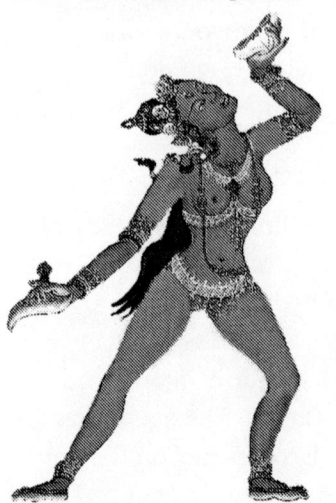

Decrees

"I AM The Light of God that Never Fails."

"I AM the inner illumination of my body, perfectly visible to my inner sight."

"I Love myself and delight in the beauty I find springing up within myself."

Maroon and Burgundy

Maroon (as well as burgundy) is a mystical application of the Red Ray. Shiva describes it as a fusing together of the Red and Green Rays. Maroon, in its fullness, represents a deep healing with the Earth and its wisdom. It allows the proper use of the Red Ray as an outpouring of the perfect timing of the Green Ray, instead of this egoic push, push, push attitude prevalent in today's workplace and social structure.

Maroon, if kept radiant, helps the deepening of the red color in one's visualization in a way that gives tremendous strength to the body. In the visualization of any of the rays, a gradual deepening of the color occurs as it becomes more tangible. However, if at any time the color loses its radiance, increase its radiance, usually by making it more transparent and a lighter shade. The process is similar to starting with a high-pitched voice and gradually bringing it to a lower tone, keeping a richness, depth, maturity and support of the higher-pitched overtones within the voice.

The full activation of this color comes from the back portion of the head, as well as from above the head. It simultaneously lights a fire of strengthening emanation from the navel and the tan tien (just below the navel). The use of the Maroon and Burgundy Rays are highly developed in some spiritual schools.

Use of the Maroon Ray can help create the a very strong, invincible feeling body. It creates a strength in the bodymind which helps hold a one-pointed concentration of focus, like a acetylene torch. It makes it easy to "key out" distractions and what you do not care about. Like any ability, this can be used positively or insensitively.

There has been a lot of "boy's club" attitude amongst those of a priestly disposition, as they extend into the Maroon Ray. Many of its members try to keep it that way, subtly blocking the entrance of the feminine from joining its little circle of light. This is not to say that they do not recognize a power within the feminine, rather it uses the feminine for its own purposes, such as to gain strength, or to exploit in some fashion, while refusing to surrender to what the feminine truly is.

A person established in the mystical strength of the Maroon Ray sometimes feels that they can make a mockery of nature, as if a law unto oneself. They can take what they want and have the strength to weather the subsequently resulting storms. Yet this is a false strength, for in the end it leaves one impoverished of the true beauty of nature. These obtrusive attempts to take of the Earth are being cleared from the Earth herself. In the clearing away of these anchors, they are not allowed to remain within the etheric fabric under our feet. This particularly affects a number of spiritual leaders, of whom it is hoped will take the next step that this occurrence asks.

Pink

Pink is a soft, creative color of a feminine nature, bringing forth a rich, thick field of ambient energy. It is of a devotional nature. It is frequently seen in the aura of yogis and people of a giving nature. When you surrender into the pink energy, your heart will float in light, bringing forth a devotion to the Divine. A few inspirational figures who carried the pink energy strongly are Mother Mary, Mary Magdalene, Jesus, Ananda Moya Ma, Tara and Paramahansa Yogananda.

Some of the wonderful qualities of a soul carrying the Pink Ray include a compassionate nature, being able to see another's point of view and a softness which carries a healing and blessing presence to all. A Pink Ray being knowingly or unknowingly values the purity of the soul above all else and naturally avoids gross people and behavior.

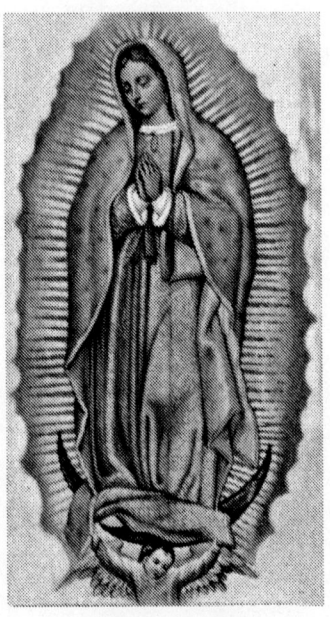

Pink is a creative and emotional energy, creating a feeling of the heart moving though the universe. Pink is very healing for the nerves. Pink has an association with the heart, spleen, a woman's ovaries, and the halo around the head: it is a component of the higher causative realms of existence. Its very open nature can bring a feeling of vulnerability, and of not having the inclination to defend itself or see fault with others.

The soft power of the Pink Ray keeps the subtle energy channels of the body pliable. Without the full development of all the rays, it is often gullible, easily led and lacks the penetrating power of discernment. The Pink Ray personality tends to make excuses and compromises for oneself and others, typically overcompensating for the behavior of others, and making statements such as, "I could not do that, it might upset so and so." Yet, when there is something they do not want to see inside of themselves, there is a tendency to manipulate others (often by being overly nice), as a way of disarming that person's penetrative stance, so that the issues are not directly confronted. Another personality issue is drawing on others for strength. It is important for a Pink Ray person to enter the stark truth of stillness, to see beyond the personality.

As in all the rays, there are those who manipulate a ray to dominate an energy field. Using the Pink Ray to manipulate the emotional energy field, especially of the opposite sex, in the long run, simply makes a lot of difficulty for the person doing it.

There are skilled manipulators who are ruthless in getting what they want through manipulating the emotional field of others by a calculated use of the mental faculties. In this way, a person can prevent others from seeing certain sensitive areas. To a true Pink Ray personality, it never occurs to them to work with this ray in such a way, so this interference is seldom seen. Many politicians use it, though unaware of the mechanics involved.

When the Pink Ray is projected from the mental faculties for the purpose of interference, it creates a subtle confusion in the energy field. From an auric perspective, this often creates a relatively crisply defined banding of pink around the head area, which holds the interfering images.[6] The band begins a number of inches out

---

[6] Do not confuse this banding with a natural occurrence of pink in the arcline (projection from the forehead). A healthy pink energy can occur in the arcline, which also at times has a crisp quality to it. This pinkness is similar to the vitality of the insides of an organ, is giving, and at least inwardly, is devotional in nature. This is much different from a calculated, unclean, ruthless, taking energy.

from the head and is usually two to eight inches thick. This is in contrast to the more surrendered and feminine use of the Pink Ray which does not have clearly defined borders, is softer, soothing and is always connected with the heart.

A person being subjected to this type of manipulation must stay on guard to constantly create a feeling of success within themselves. They must subtly redefine all energies in their auric field with that crisp, clear feeling of the heart living in Perfection.

Do not let this put you off using pink in the head centers and above, as this is a very valuable and necessary development. Just be sure to keep the purity, sincerity, and heart connection; the Pink Ray will greatly serve you in bringing forth feeling into manifestation. Combining gold with your pink attunement gives greater confidence. Blue keeps everything on track and aligned. Blue is a very good color for Pink Ray types to embrace.

There is a very conscious radiance of the Pink Ray on the sixth dimension emanated forth by various Masters on the planet Venus. Those who ground this benefit from a refined consciousness that does not carry some of the more dense karmas within our solar system.

Decrees

"I AM the blessing presence."

"I AM the illumined mind radiating in the heart of all God's children."

"I AM the forgiveness of all unenlightened activity."

Orange

The Orange Ray is a bright, happy, sensual, fluid, ecstatic, transformational presence that holds deep mystic truths. Of course, we are talking of an activated, bright, sunshine-like Orange Ray. As a tremendously creative, limitless ecstasy, you can telescope inwardly upon it into your Divine Presence as a field of infinitely bright whiteness. It connects you directly to the unlimited solar radiance that is the bliss of creation. Great cosmic beings wield the Orange Ray as a transformational power. Emotional manifestation of desires can occur through its ecstasy and transcending power. This wonderfully ecstatic and refreshing ray has a great cosmic heritage.

The Orange Ray gives a lot of freedom, because it contains a direct connection to the tremendous freedom inherent in the flame of existence. If a person takes license to qualify this sense of freedom from the lower self, he or she creates distortions and muddies its brilliance. This results in a rebellious attitude and resistance to one's own perfection of light.

Care is needed when first meditating on this ray. Its activation will tend to focus attention in the second chakra and genitals, stimulating erotic feelings, passions and all sorts of images. The practitioner works with this energy by constantly circulating its stimulation into the upper centers. Valuable tools include pranayama, visualization, yoga sets, and deep meditation upon your formless essence. As the practitioner makes significant breakthroughs with their emotional healing, the sexual current originating from the genitals begins to fuse directly into the upward movement of the spinal current and fusion channel.

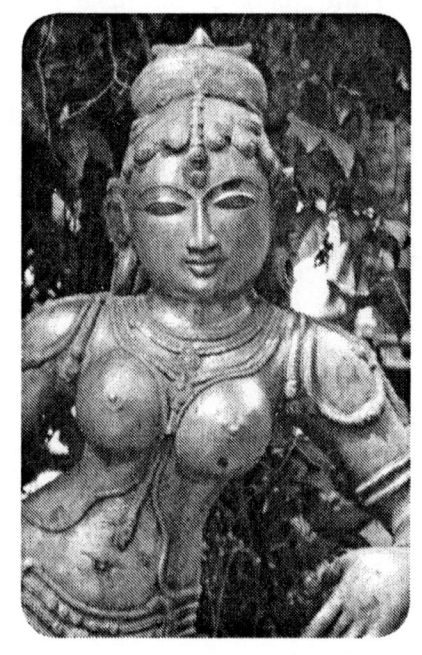

As this fusion continues, energy is no longer seen as sexual; it is just energy, so it is naturally transformed as part of a whole-body-presence directed by inner clarity—your I AM Presence. When you have totally elevated your use of the Orange Ray from a personal-emotional-sexual orientation into its cosmic ecstasy, this ray becomes widespread in its distribution through the body, drawing in universal energy as nectar.

The Orange Ray helps emotionally to awaken the heart and clear obstructions along the channels, particularly along the spine. It can become inwardly visible in awakening a number of different centers in the body, bringing a seductive feeling of a great outpouring of mystery. Not that it is a mystery, rather the emotional feeling of ecstasy can give the feeling that life contains so much more than most grant it.

Visualize yourself entering an orange sphere of light and give yourself into its transforming joy. The analytical mind is totally dissolved; one laughs for no reason at all! You know the feeling of freedom—bliss is the true freedom. You realize that you have such great freedom, no one is telling you what you can or cannot do, you just are. In this, the only limit to the ecstasy is the degree to which you can expand to become it. In the center of this orange lightning, telescoping deeper and deeper is a cosmic white light of truth, direct from the truth of your soul, beyond all outer qualification. With nothing else to do, this truth becomes your life.

In the 1800's and early 1900's a wave of Masters who were expert in the Orange Ray came forth upon this planet to do deep transformational work upon the collective psyche, preparing it for the new age dawning upon humanity. Much of this work was not outwardly recognized. Some of these beings include Lahiri Mahasaya (Mahavatar BabaJi's principle disciple at that time), Sri Yukteswar, Sarada Devi (Ramakrishna's Twin Ray and consort), Nityananda (the Guru of Muktananda), Ramana Maharshi of South India, Mahatma Ghandi, Sri Aurobindo and his Twin Ray who was simply called "The Mother" by her devotees.

The Beloved Master Lantro (also known as Milarepa) is particularly strong on the Orange Ray, as is Lord Meru.

The cosmic being Shiva is a Lord of the Orange Ray for our system. He has also been referred to as the Venusian being, Serapis. His great love for the Himalayan Mountains has brought forth his presence into the very atoms of its mighty ranges. He has a particularly active interest in America and is working to remove the spiritual distortions so prevalent, that this land may come forth unhindered in its great providence as a place radiating the necessary feeling of what it means to be purely in your Individualized God Presence.

There is a widespread feeling in the United States that this land is like a clean slate upon which a new beginning rose up from the heavily polluted psychic field of Europe. While this definitely has a truth, it is ignorant of the great land that America is; she is very sacred and ancient, containing hidden treasures within her atoms. The soul remembrance of this land is being more and more being activated in the subtle levels, which will come forth in the feelings of many individuals.

Having traveled broadly, I experience that even with its many problems, America is forging ahead as a cutting-edge in bringing forth the new spirituality for the awakened humanity of our planet. This new spirituality is not based on old structures, but on the intuitive light of the Individualized God Presence. Penetrating into the Radiant depth of your own Presence is the doorway into awakening into the ecstatic reality of the Oneness. Being in the Oneness is not in any way a loss of individuality—just the opposite, for to remain conscious in such a family, you must find the wonder of your own Light. The Orange Ray brings forth the permission, the cellular freedom to ignite the feeling of the Divine intimately at work, in a play of magnificent proportions.

Through enough deep, liberating meditation, the ecstatic creative energy is felt everywhere in the body and originates from above as well. The predominately Orange Ray personality will use the tremendous creative freedom felt from the Orange Ray to rebel against what are felt as restrictions from society; this will continue until this personality stops looking outwardly and recognizing instead, the infinite as the source of beautiful and ecstatic occurrence. Release your attention into cosmic consciousness and transformative service.

Orange is a ray of transmutation and of ecstatic creation. It is sensual, earthy, mystical, radiant, and brings forth beauty, strength and stability. Orange is a color of the soil and may be thought of as the soil of the body. If your soil is strong, you will be strong. If it is weak then you cannot ground the full voltage of the spirit. Thus orange is a quality that we can use to transmute the cellular structure of our bodies, quickening and raising their vibration.

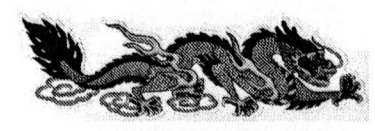

Within the Devic kingdom, the Naga spirits, make great use of the Orange Ray (of course, they are not limited only to this ray). This is primarily because of the fluid-watery quality within the Naga kingdom. Nagas live very much in, although not exclusively limited to, the water element; think of waterfalls, pools, sensuous experiences. They have a lot of psychic sensitivity and can affect this within people. In the physical, Nagas sometimes ground through snakes, although it is not correct to think of them as reptiles. The Nagas attune to the kundalini flows within the earth, and can affect these flows as well. Some Nagas advance into becoming dragons,[7] which is a very high spiritual achievement, far beyond what most humans can conceive of.

---

[7] Most people have a mistaken view of what dragons are. Dragons are an aspect of the devic kingdom that was active long before human kind appeared on the earth. They are buddhic beings, some of whom are adepts and masters at the highest levels of creation, working deeply within the earth. Probably the best way to think of the dragons is as the kundalini flows of the earth, for they embody upon these flows, and the more advanced ones create them as well. Each type of energy has a kind of subtle fragrance, like a subtle mist. A water dragon is a dragon that embodies upon an essence of water, a fire dragon embodies up an essence of fire, a space dragon embodies upon the nectars of space. The dragons are often responsible for creating a lot of the topographies and elemental energetic supports on the earth, around which countries and cultures form.

Dragons are hypersensitive by nature, as is any being that embodies dominantly upon an elemental energy. They work in the bigger picture, and can clear large amounts of blockages created through unconsciousness. As they once again take a more active role influencing the activities on the surface of the earth, and helping the Devic kingdom regain its rightful respect, this will result in widespread subtle changes, including cleansings and a change of power.

Some people easily effect, and are affected by, the Nagas. Taking this symbiosis too far, there are those, either consciously or unconsciously, who capture the psychic energy of a Naga spirit into their own subtle nervous system. This forced binding, often initially obtained through covert seduction, is a gross misuse of energy, and while it gives experience to both parties, there is usually a huge kickback down the line. This occurs more often than realized, particularly within shamanistically-orientated individuals, those who are seeking psychic powers, and through heavy misuse of sexual energy. This seldom gives a pure view of the Naga realms themselves; it is like raping a woman and expecting the relationship to be of any value. Psychedelic drugs have the potential to open people into the psychic sensitivity of the Naga world; however, this is often weakening to the body (and seldom gives the correct perspective).

From another angle, there are also immature Naga spirits who will draw on excess sexual energy, often to the detriment of the human who does not know better. Once you purify and awaken the back of the head, you are in command of the energy. The back of the head is an important center within the Orange Ray. It is important in opening it up, that you do so in a pure way, otherwise you will simply be playing in a lower astral field of unfulfilled desires and emotions, which makes unending difficulties in your life. Drugs are probably the biggest obstacle in opening up this energy correctly, with a close second being the misuse of feminine energy. If these are issues for you, then take care of this first, before you attempt to awaken in the back of the head. Otherwise, these tendencies will continue to want control, and it is unlikely you will proceed correctly.

Some Kriya Yogis use Orange to help transmute their bodies into light. This involves the buddhic application of the Orange Ray to elevate the very atoms of the body to a higher frequency. Orange always works with other qualities, just as the soil serves the plants that grow in it. Orange, when unbridled, brings the capacity for change.

Orange consumes and creates at the same time. Initially work with this quality by anchoring it several inches up from the base of the spine, where it finds a resonance with the sexual energy. Then fill the heart and the whole body with a bright and extremely lively orange. As it moves upwards, I find that orange creates the feeling of being earthy in the vastness of outer space, which is an ecstatic feeling. After purifying the second chakra, the Orange Ray does not need to be anchored through the lower spine, but simply through the free attention of consciousness.

A bright, free visualization of the Orange Ray is great for purifying the lymph in the body. This clear fluid plays an important spiritual function for the adept, as it becomes a "second semen." Purified lymph is a vessel to receive cosmic electricity, store it and circulate this vitality throughout the body. Purification of the lymph goes hand-in-hand with cleansing of the bone marrow, tendons and particularly the joints.

Orange is a mystical color, which in its purity hints of hidden mysteries, of the nature of creation, all within a framework of Love of the Divine. Yet it is only a hint, as it needs the fuller picture for its satisfaction. It is not by chance that many swamis wear orange, as one needs strong roots to fly high; orange helps in this grounding. An advanced Yogi or Yogini may discover its awakening in the heart, which brings an ecstatic, internal dance beyond description. Advanced Yogis use the Orange Ray to help purify collective karmas.

The Orange Ray, if not developed in balance with the other colors and through internal recognition of divinity, brings forth an obvious impulsive nature and more subtle tendencies of possessiveness and pride. This impulsive nature can result in a karmic trail left behind, like yesterday's lunch. In time, this catches up with us, and we are asked to develop other aspects.

An Orange Ray personality has to be careful in regards to excess and addictions, as the saying goes, "sex, drugs, and rock n' roll." While their transformative capacity generally allows a greater capacity of excess, still it becomes a serious problem in regards to spiritual practice, from the side affects of abuse, and because it prevents a stabilization of higher awareness.

When orange becomes dull, it leads to an earthy stuckness and covert activity. While outwardly accepting of people, it subtly blocks free movement of higher energy, and a depressive attitude can result. While there can be many reasons for swings between happy and depressive moods, for an Orange Ray personality on the spiritual path, this often indicates a need for development on other rays, such as green, blue, and violet. The solution will take a committed long-term dedication to spiritual application. Kriya practice is important. Release the need to have things your way, not just outwardly, but also inwardly; otherwise, a "spoiled brat" can result. There is often a secret fascination with psychic phenomena.

Unfortunately, some personalities use the Orange Ray as a qualification of mysticism and magnetism operating through a combination of intellectual and psychic shamanism. In reality, such an "expert" dilutes the spiritual path, creating a muddy, polluted orange color in the energy field, which can only be washed away by embracing the pure, tangible presence of higher radiance.

Orange has the capacity to stimulate your subconscious mind; it can bring forth a flood or swirl of images. If a person is not inwardly clean and of a meditative mind, then this can lead to a loss of focus and grounding. Oddly, the loss of grounding is the opposite of what this color brings to an integrated personality.

A predominant Orange Ray person truly benefits from a competent spiritual teacher, who can show, through transmission and beingness, the intricate balance of personality and impersonality necessary to bring growth on this ray. It is also important for predominant Orange Ray beings to discipline themselves, including following through with an intention, to bring forth development on the other rays.

To clear distortions of the Orange Ray, recognize your light as a manifestation of the Oneness, so there is nothing to rebel against. Simultaneously, everything in your life is a result of your own creation, thus you must own the responsibility.

Decrees

"I AM the fulfillment of all that I desire."

"I AM the victorious presence reclaiming every cell of my body temple."

"I AM Bliss."

Emerald Green

The Green Ray holds dominion over the terrestrial world in the same way that the Blue Ray feels its home in cosmic truth. The Green Ray expression does not feel truly comfortable until it knows that all the rays are given their due expression and acknowledgment. Thus, the Green Ray is involved in emotional healing and harmony.

The Green Ray involves connectivity—connectivity of words such as in poetry and linguistic skills, connectivity of sound as in music, imaging of space as in art, in science through understanding, and spatial connectivity of the body to elevate it in light.

Balance, harmony, love, electromagnetic presence, penetration, peace, stillness within form, compassion, integration, neutrality, musical ability and linguistic skill are all Green Ray qualities. Green is a color of the heart and of nature. Science seeks to understand the relationship and connectivity of creation. This brings an interesting observation, that science may be explored in modern days with the intellect, but it is the stillness and connectivity which in poignant moments brings forth understanding.

Green stimulates the pineal gland, opening into a greater relationship with the cosmos. Green helps integrate new experiences and your environment. Being able to integrate experience results in a healthy, disease-free embodiment with strong nerves. Green, in its harmonizing quality, is a color of the liver energy and may be visualized there with great benefit. Green foods strengthen the heart, nerves, and liver. There is a natural connection of the Green Ray with the movement of the air element.

The Green Ray holds an important key for the next step for humanity's evolution into the heart, a consciousness aware of the inter-connectivity of all life and the quickening of the body's molecular structure.

Green accentuates a feeling of the love, peace, and beauty of harmony. In its purity, the heart is the first ascending center of consciousness established above judgment. The heart is an ever-present sanctuary where you can dissolve the clatter of the mind into beingness. It is a home base from which to learn of the quiet way. In this classroom, one learns how to forge ahead in the higher realms by traveling deeper within the heart.

The Green Ray is particularly adept at linguistics, poetry, and expressing itself through writing. Writing a journal or speaking in depth with others helps your Green Ray development. For this to be potent, however, it must include deep, penetrating meditation to bring forth insight from the great silence of your being, for the science of interconnectivity that the Green Ray knows is deep. No matter how well the trusses on a bridge are constructed, if the whole structure is not connected firmly to bedrock, i.e., based on truth, then it will simply crumble in the face of testing weather. Analogy is a tool often used on the Green Ray.

Distortion on the Green Ray creates distortion of time and space and modifies inherent perfection into disharmony by inappropriately pushing or avoiding the timing of situations. This lack of higher trust brings forth covertly hidden self-image problems, jealousy, and looking outside of yourself for the answers. It can be very subtle, especially when hidden behind a charismatic outer show.

Self-correction requires feeling the harmony of perfection and all the rays in harmony. Distortion of the Green Ray often compels the more outwardly visible Gold Ray into misqualification of will power. This deception can be very good at covering its tracks; thus, a person doing so in using the Green Ray often ends up deceiving him or her self.

This can result in trying to impose your own timing onto another. Again, to clear distortions on any ray, all the rays must be brought forth. The Blue Ray, if held as a central point of command, as a bright, radiant light in the center of inner awareness, can bring forth the conflicts of the outer personality and create the openings for deeper alignment into the cosmic perfection.

In the process of clearing these distortions, I have found it extremely helpful to feel that the fabric of terrestrial space is made of a beautiful, deep, emerald green light containing within it a sense of perfect connectivity and timing. Any ripples of congestion on this perfect fabric are the result of egoic contractions. I use the penetrating power of my 'I AM' Presence to see what is behind those ripples and bring it to the clear brightness of the green fabric. This green is a combination of deep emerald-green with a bright, translucent clear light that shows it is connected to the higher causal planes of existence. This has a greater capacity of bringing forth a quickening of perfection.

There is a tendency of the Green Ray personality to place the power in things outside of themselves. Their natural ability of connectivity and allowance makes the arts of astrology, I-ching, tarot cards, divination in general, and muscle testing for psychic answers attractive. Yet this fascination can covertly become a play in the shadows and extremely disempowering. An element of uncertainty is always present, and in this dualistic mindset, the doors are open for all sorts of confusion. This is in exact opposition to the feeling necessary to effectively apply your I AM Presence as the governing force of your world, the ability to go direct and receive every answer you need.

The heart is more than human feeling. This is a partial opening of the heart, but it must open further to Divine Wisdom, which always brings forth a blissful feeling with it that is unmistakable. The heart is connected above the head, then above that to its Divine source within the heart[8] into ever-opening circles of Love and Perfection, which can see, be fearless, and remain at peace in the higher knowingness of Perfection.

A person who has not surrendered into the full opening of the heart must guard themselves from jealousy, subtle manipulation of circumstances, lack of commitment and a very tricky level of deceptive dishonesty of which they may not even be aware. All this comes from an inner battle between the soul knowing the potential of this ray and the psychic capacities of the ray operating within a heart closed to the higher wisdom presence. This scenario makes it very difficult for the kundalini to rise and stay at the level of the heart, as the cleverness of the person inadvertently brings it back down. The only way out is through using the tremendous courage inherent within this ray to remain humble, while practicing a strong sadhana and being one-hundred percent honest with yourself.

[8] This is a reference to the light beyond the light, of which the point way above the head is a doorway. This same doorway is in the center of the heart, and ultimately in every point of creation.

To understand the power of the Green Ray in regards to healing and precipitation, meditate upon the feeling of magnetic attraction and repulsion. Get in touch with the feeling of these forces.

Now visualize a cloud of electrons swirling around the nucleus of an atom. The cloud of electrons makes an indescribable inner sound. Get in touch with this sound as an inner radiation, and then connect it with the Green Ray. As you feel this quality in the atoms you are visualizing, let this song resonate over the entire body.

The song takes voice through a resonance of creation, corresponding to the depth and connectivity of your visualization, i.e., how much it penetrates through the subtle dimensions into observable reality. By penetrating into the feeling of the Green Ray and changing the octave of this song, you are able to change the vibrational rate of the electrons in your body, thus changing the dimension in which your body exists. When mastered, the feeling becomes so smooth that it feels as natural as walking after standing still.

There is another aspect of the feeling-connectivity of the Green Ray that helps to heal the body. On a basic physical level, what is it that holds up a muscle, keeps a muscle taut, or lets it sag? What is it that brings a feeling of everything suspended and held in just the right space in the body, or else lacking vitality? While this can be addressed on many levels, in the end it all comes down to the electrical charge present on a molecular and atomic level of the body. An inner mastery of the Green Ray can help to restore the balance and proper relationship of every atom molecule, cell, and area of the body in relation to every other part of the body. Again, this is an inner song of resonance within the feeling of perfection inherent in your I AM Presence.

Tara is a highly advanced Master of Green Ray, as is Hilarion (Guru Nanak).

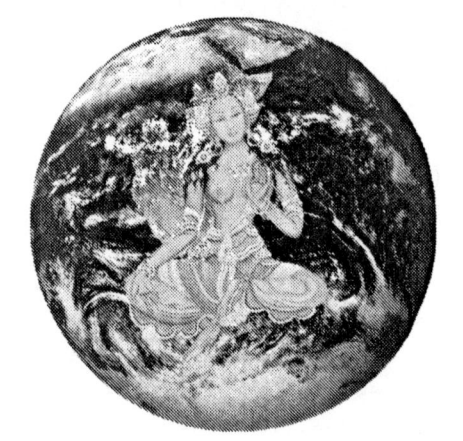

Decrees

"I AM the perfect timing of all manifestations within the I AM Presence."

"I AM the Presence on guard, allowing no disruptive forces to enter this body temple."

"I AM the earth. The earth is my body."

Violet

The Violet Ray is a high level of pranic attainment and has an amazing ability to qualify and thus change conditions within the world and ourselves.

The Violet Ray is often used for purification and protection. Meditate with it at the third eye, within the spine, within the body as a whole, and permeating the space in which you reside.

An intense attunement with the Violet Flame brings forth great richness, eloquence, and a loving elevation. Violet is the fusing of the red and Blue Rays, action, and wisdom as one expression. The Violet Flame gains its strength from the light above the head, bringing freedom from all outer circumstances not of this light. It requires a firm commitment to the light as your tangible source of support through all difficulties. It gives forth the wonderful eloquence and practical wisdom contained within it that constantly echoes forth the feeling of living in the heart-quality of Oneness. Leading visionaries in society often work on the Violet Ray.

The Violet Ray has a way of being ahead of its time, although with the increased support from within the earth for its activities, this is becoming less and less of an issue. This brings forth another, seldom understood, aspect of this ray, which is how it works deeply within the earth to bring about change, from the inside out.

Because this ray has long been associated with bringing forth greater definition of the individual, it is often championed as a support for individualistic cultures such as the United States, or past cultures such as Atlantis. While there is some truth in this, there is a better way to view this. The Violet Ray emphasizes the individual because of its gifts of alchemical transformation, which requires a knowingness of self. However, its true level of alchemy cannot occur in an individual who cannot blend beyond their self. It is just as important to be beyond individuality, as it is to be defined as an individual, if you wish to work in the true light of this ray. Its emphasis on individuality is another way of saying that you cannot progress in the tantras if you are bound to social consciousness.

Individuals with a predominant Violet Ray often are of a refined and sensitive nature. When the Violet Ray becomes the sole habit of an individual, then arrogance can easily set in. A fascination with subtle phenomena for its own sake brings us into a phenomenal world while still distant from the deeper truths of reality.

To clear distortions of this ray, you must also be clear and vital on the Red and Blue Rays. You have to mature through resistance in the form of rebellion or an overly intellectual nature. Such distortion can display itself as idealism without the ability to penetrate into the details of reality. As conflicts on the Red and Blue Rays are healed, then the Violet Flame can come out in its full strength, which is more than just red and blue together. Violet is a very high frequency possessing the ability to penetrate deeply into its environment, hold a purifying presence, and brings forth a greater reality. An example of a person with a strong Violet Ray out of balance is a high strung personality who tends to run away with themselves, leaving a trail of unfinished karmas.

You must be beyond reaction and beyond polarization to distorted energy, to experience and fully acknowledge your inner God Flame as your living, breathing, and very real Presence of Life. Activation of the eighth and ninth chakras above the head and their grounding into the physical body is necessary to clear the subtle distortions contained within these higher centers.

Applying the purifying power of the Violet Flame prepares the outer self to receive and thus awaken to the inner reality.

For a supreme teaching of the Violet Ray, read the books by Godfre' Ray King (a pen name for Guy Ballard) written in the 1930's in which he describes his personal training with Saint Germain. In my opinion, the first three books of this series (the green books published by the Saint Germain Press) are some of the highest and most elevating words ever written in the English language. I highly recommend that you read them.

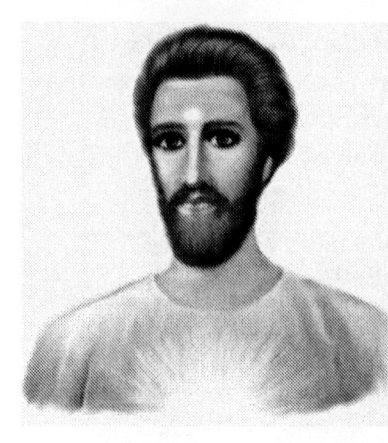

They have a power of transmission because the aura of the books are directly connected to the radiant field of the Masters. If read with an open mind and pure heart, these books bring forth the feeling radiations behind the experiences talked about, helping you with your own application of the teachings.

This type of connectivity is in itself an example of the eloquence of the Violet Flame, which has so much potential for bringing humanity quickly to another level of existence. While simple in acknowledgment, the depth of penetration required to understand and wield the power behind the omnipotent flame of your Presence requires an earnest and committed application to bring forth.

The Violet Flame is often the last ray to be taught, because it requires a mature soul to grasp that, "The fullness of the individual and awakening into Oneness are the same thing."

The Violet Ray is magical, transforming, and somewhat elusive at times in definition, yet elegantly expressive, honest, and present. It expresses itself in a sensitive royalty; if it was not for its frank humility, it could be mistaken as arrogant in its charisma. The Violet Ray does not compromise the truth. It is a ray of vision, dancing between formlessness and form. It transforms existence, opens the intuition to truth and makes life an art and dance of essence into form. The Violet Flame is alchemical in nature. It is very close to the Devic kingdom and its understandings, revealing the key to unlock the secrets of matter in consciousness.

There are those who misuse the Violet Ray, turning it into a kind of sticky substance, more dull in color. This is then used as a carrier for their desires. One of the qualities of this kind of etheric substance is that it must shut down certain higher faculties for it to work. For example, you may feel a pressure in your temples, as if someone is trying to place a lid on the top of your head. The solution is to bring forth an intensely bright and high-pitched application of the Violet Flame. For those who have the purity, soft lavender applied with a devic elevation, can easily override the misuse of the Violet Flame. It is a general principal that a higher frequency of a ray will dissolve the power of that ray when misused. This will only work if the person bringing forth that application is free of karmic entanglement and polarity with the being(s) who are misqualifying the ray.

A further, more subtle misuse of the Violet Flame occurs through subtle mental activity. A typical example is projecting desires in the buddhic realms and giving them the force of a decree, without truly understanding the light beyond the light and ourselves beyond personality. This activity often occurs on the Silver Ray and uses the Violet Flame as a means of effect. The solution is to bring back the brilliance of the Silver Ray from pure source, which then dissolves the subtle fabrics of support wrongly created.

Interestingly, two of the countries perhaps most significant to the Violet Flame, China and the United States, outwardly appear very different. Of course, the emphasis of the individual in the United States makes a good support for the Violet Flame. In China, the incredible excellence and high achievements within this society, particularly in the alchemical arts, also creates a wonderful support of the Violet Flame. In addition, the Violet Flame, as a spiritual quality, has long been outwardly recognized as a high achievement in China.

Freedom, Divinity, Sensitivity and Transformation in returning to the Self as the cause of creation are all aspects of the Violet Ray. Within the tantric mandala of the Ascended Masters, Saint Germain is often invoked and felt as the Lord and overseer of this ray.

Decrees

"I AM all that I wish to be and manifest."

"I AM the clear path to the Beloved Ascended Masters."

"Oh Mighty Violet Flame, enter this body temple of my Presence and purify it forever of all impurities, limitations and unenlightened memories."

"I AM my I AM Presence."

The White Light

White light is the "earth of heaven." Its use facilitates creation of nectar, and thus strengthens the body. The cosmic quality of white light combined with its tangibility helps greatly in purification, nourishment, and refinement. We open up, tangibly, to a greater dimension of ourselves.

Meditating on the white light in the crown center can create an opening for a transmission of multi-colored nectar-light that appears as flashes of all the different colors together descending into the body. The effects are beyond description, other than to say, when properly received, this elevates the frequency of the entire body into light.

Developing nectar within the body will forever remove any doubt as to the effectiveness of spiritual practices, and is something that anyone, who keeps their practice alive and potent over time, can achieve. Nectar is a magical substance both physical and ethereal, that is, it exists in full presence in both realties. As such, it bridges the worlds into a continuum.

The seminal fluids and essences (of both men and woman) are the beginnings of nectar. These fluids help bridge the gap for the soul to take birth into physicality. In daily life, they firm the mind and emotions by helping to ground our soul into the body. Through yogic practice, we refine these nectars and bring them into the upper centers. We then effortlessly absorb our mind into the sensations and vistas of our soul and we have the physiological support of the body in doing so. In places such as the back of the head, also called the "mouth of God," we can use these nectars to seduce very fine nectar-essences, not normally of this body, to precipitate into it. As they do so, they join with the nectars you have already refined, thus preventing these incredibly fine substances from evaporating. Within these breathless-nectars[9], you will know yourself in essence beyond the limiting confines of the body.

---

[9] Breathless, because they are not born of the physical breath or the substances moved by subtle activity of the physical breath, such as seminal fluids. They are also termed breathless, because as your attention becomes absorbed into them, your physical breath tends to disappear. You are sourcing yourself from a very deep place.

White, as a color, is almost synonymous with the word, "light." White light can be used anywhere in the body, but first visualizing it in the crown, back of the head, or the thymus, gives it a better capacity to further work anywhere in the body as needed. This also helps open you to realities beyond your immediate personality.

By visualizing white light above the head, you can activate the eighth center and bring a greater tangibility to your awareness. This visualization will initiate purification, provided you stay with the essence of the light rather than becoming caught in the images of purification.

Some members of the Devic Kingdom use a luscious, brilliant, and at the same time soft, white light as their life force and will heal others through this light. In addition, there is a particular class of beings within the earth, seldom connected with other than by adepts, who use this light to do a specialized, secret work for the earth.

White, as an earth color, strengthens and gives substance wherever it is used. It finds a home, whether visualized in the physical aspects of the body, its chakras and channels, or in the buddhic realms—helping to birth form into being. Immersing yourself in a thick tube of brilliant white originating from above your head, and while sustaining that, bring forth a radiant image of yourself in the center of the head. After sitting with this for some time, extend it to your body as a whole, then back again into the center of the head. The white light can help you get in touch, tangibly, with your subtle body.

Another practice is to visualize a white, five-pointed star in the third eye. Visualize this under the skin, not in front, and smaller rather than big, perhaps a quarter-inch in size is best. Within the whiteness of the five-pointed star, give it a transparent, beyond-everything quality, telescoping from infinity into this form. After you have stabilized this image and its qualities, become aware of the various parts of the face and forehead. Visualize one or more of the tips of the five pointed star stretching out to connect with a particular point on your face, such as the corner of your eye, a crease on your face, etc. Keep the same omnisciently powerful quality of the white, somewhat-transparent light through that ray from the tip of the star. As it connects to this part of your face, feel the muscles, the tissues, the bone underneath responding and rejuvenating, becoming filled with youthful light. Stay with each area for some time. When you are accomplished at this, then extend the tip(s) of the star to anywhere on the body.

A good way to work with white light is to first cultivate it at the third eye, by breathing in a sensuous white mist that gradual forms a liquid-light. This can take a few weeks or months of consistent application. To better support this, you may want to first breathe up and down your spine and open up the back of the head. When you actually feel a sense of space within your third eye, like a small cave perfumed by the sense of liquid white light, center within that wonderful feeling as a very small brilliant point of presence. The purpose of starting with the third eye is to gain a greater activation within this light. Next, drop down deep into the chest and visualize a soft white light. This can either be in the area of the heart, or the thymus. It is important to keep the visualization and its resultant energy soft and alive. Do not synchronize it with the breath at all. That is, it does not matter if you are inhaling or exhaling, the light stays the same regardless. It will create a presence that will stay with you after your formal sitting. While the light may start as three or four inches across in size, do not focus on giving it an exact shape; just allow it gradually to build in presence and awareness. As it does, feel it spreading through the chest, into the arms, and throughout the body. Do not use external will power to do this visualization; otherwise, you could disrupt the balance of the physical heart, which is dangerous. It must be kept soft and, from within that softness strength is drawn.

In this practice, you are attuning the physical tissues to respond to and receive this light. Through this simple act, you are creating a bridge from the invisible realm of subtle light into a tangible act, such as releasing tension in a muscle and energizing it. If in the practice of the previous paragraph, you are in your head, visualizing this presence in your chest, then that is not it. You have to drop your center of focus down into the area you which to center within. There is the feeling that you are looking out from within that place, not looking down into it from the head.

For all of the above practices you will greatly benefit by invoking the presence of various Devic Masters to help you. Go for walks in nature. Make little offerings of food and thanks. Imagine yourself going into the earth, give thanks, and ask for help. Without this blessing and opening, your practice will not progress far into the true inner understanding.

Devas are those who consciously work within the etheric fabric of creation in awareness and honoring of the oneness of all creation. By right of this application and attunement, the Devas not only work in this fabric, but they are the consciousness of the underlying etheric fabric itself without which, literally, none of us could exist. Therefore, in a very real way, we are all from the devic reality, although when steeped in separation, we forget this. From the perspective of the higher realms, in all of creation there is nothing else other than Devas, nor can there be, for it is manifestation itself. Many kingdoms come out of this, such as legions of Angels, plant, mineral, animal and human kingdoms, not to mention countless others not known to most two-leggeds. Yet for the most part, when reference is made to the devic kingdom, it is to the masterful beings within the earth (and cosmos), invisible to most people, who live and work within the greater good. Many of these beings are referred to as angels.

White is associated with purity. However, I have also seen fifth-dimensional demons clothed in bodies of a chalky-white astral light. It is not just the color white, but the feeling within it that is important. Make sure it contains the purity of the infinitude behind it, the inherent perfection of your source, the stainless attribute of truth. Call it forth as a brilliant, scintillating, alive light in which every ray can come forth at any second as a youthful and eternal quality. There is a moist quality, not a dry one with it. Any necessary color can come out of it and dissolve back into it.

An excellent practice is to visualize the bones as made of white light with a tinge of gold. However, do not feel that you need to limit it only to the bones. Always qualify this light as having great strength, sweetness, a warmness or pleasant temperature, and a youthful quality. If visualizing the bones as white, make sure you include the feeling of breathing prana easily into the bone. Feel the bright red blood in the center of the bone marrow.

Aspects of your visualization to help this qualification would be to feel your face as youthful, of a sweet disposition and radiant. You can imagine holding a bone in your hand and testing it, through various imaginations, to show its incredible strength. Make sure that you qualify it with a strength that makes it unbreakable, even giving a sense of magnetic force through the bone of such strength that it repels any destructive force away from it. Practice breathing energy into the bones, then holding the breath while you concentrate the prana. As you slowly exhale, keep the energy in and around the bones, creating warmth.

Do not let your visualization of the white light take on a chalky, cold, removed sensation. If you do so, you may easily find yourself attuning to some of the more polluted astral realms and a sense of decay. Sometimes images come forth clothed in this type of light as you are purifying yourself or your environment. These images are disconnected remnants of past activity as remembered in your tissues or in the tissues of the earth, or they are discarnate spirits, like ghosts, that are not able to bring the warmer earth energies into their constitution.

White is an excellent color to accentuate the pure visualization of another color, giving strength to that color. You can use the white light hand-in-hand with the Violet Flame in purification of hidden and troublesome energies latching onto your emotional and subtle bodies. In meditating with a pure white light, discordant energies more easily stand out. It is then easier to keep a focus of the Violet Flame through the area, consuming the images; in the whiteness there is nowhere for them to hide. The white light also enhances the brightness and depth of the Violet Flame you bring forth.

A bright, fun, sensuous, and mystic orange, works very closely with the white light. You can meditate on this kind of orange light and feel that it is originating out of a white light in the center of it. If your life is getting too drab, too serious, and not blissful enough, then meditate on the orange and white light. Let it make you laugh more.

By first meditating on white throughout the body, you will feel the richness of a king so close that you may just expect a drop of gold to materialize in your hand. Remember to give it a sweet, youthful,

Soul Development through the Rays of Light 167

strong, soft and warm quality. Then bring forth a golden light in your hands, in your heart, or wherever your attention is focused.

By visualizing white and green, you adjust the space that everything in you body takes, i.e., you correct the magnetic web of the body that holds everything in its proper place. In this type of meditation, keep the colors distinct, yet allow them to overlap and come out of each other, moving in the same harmony. When finished, you may like to experiment and blend the various colors into one new color.

While the mind alone can bring forth, and work with, the various colors as you move them through the body or visualize something, it is a tremendous assistance to remember the breath. You can either actively use the breath by charging it with various colors and attributes and then directing the breath as desired, or else you can keep a continual deep breath going on in the background. Feel it open the inner space of the body, bringing in aliveness and alertness into the cells of the body.

Decrees

"I AM my subtle body within the Light I AM."

"I AM precipitating nectars nourishing this body."

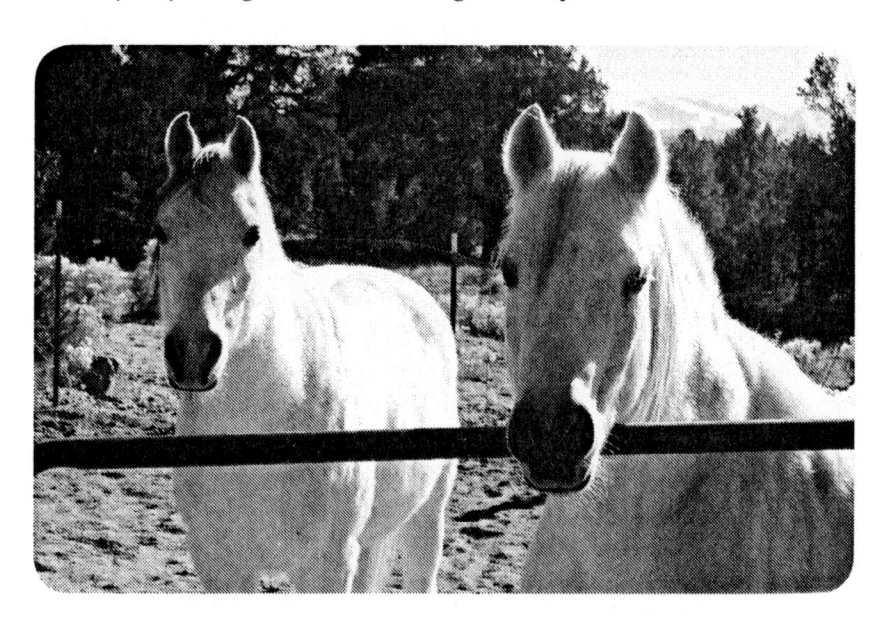

Silver

The Silver Ray is a cosmic consciousness that can be used to bridge the buddhic realms into the physical. Adepts use this nectar light to aid in precipitation, and as a very fine energy within the body.

For a person whose existence is predominantly within a karmic perspective the Silver Ray does not have any physiological grounding within the body at all. In contrast, the more common rays all support everyday thought processes, emotions, and energetic workings of the body. Thus, at first working with the Silver Ray can be quite slippery to understand. If you bring it deep enough, your body will gradually adapt to it through its outpourings within the chakras.

Most people initially connect to the Silver Ray above the head and keep it there or in the head. As such, it is like an invisible high voltage electrical quality that can create dryness around the head, headaches and sharpness in your disposition. Pressure in the head and headaches are a common side effect of strong Silver Ray activity, although there are ways to work with the energy so this does not occur.

When you can bring this ray deeper into the body, it can then stimulate your various elemental qualities in more of a balance. The proper place to ground this ray is through the central channel gradually outwards, through blending with the body's nectar. Trying to ground it first through the outer energy structure, if done too intensely, can be dangerous to your health and cause sickness that is not easy to cure, except through rest and dissolving the outer creations of your mind while going deeper within.

From within the central channel, the natural places to first bring out this ray are the sexual, thymus, and throat centers. From these places, keep it allied with a blue or white-liquid quality. From within the navel area it can be used as a cosmic fire brilliant with visionary ability. This fire includes an elemental balance with the water and spatial qualities, resulting in a coolness and warmth at the same time.

The Silver Ray brings greater telepathic awareness and ability of projection. It is a ray of manifestation and can work with the energy of manifestation beyond normal confines of space and time.

Because of its ability to bridge the gap from the buddhic to the physical experience, this can include direct precipitation.

The Silver Ray helps greatly in regeneration of the body. As you gain mastery with this ray, you will remain strong while simultaneously transparent. This is an advanced activity, just short of displaying physically tangible siddhas.

When working with, receiving, or strongly experiencing the Silver Ray, you may find karmic limitations of your life being blown apart. This includes anything in your life that you know is holding back your spiritual movement, which you just accept anyway. Examples would be a stuck marriage, wrong job, limiting likes and dislikes, attachments, and difficulties of your disposition. On top of this, there will be a part of you that does not care that your life is falling apart. You can even develop a flippant attitude, seeing yourself in a different frame of reference than most people. While this, at times, can be a great gift, be careful not to throw the baby out with the bath water. As this ray is formed from within your higher energy body, it has little respect for limitations that are going to hold you back. Thus, you must be ready for and accept change (for the better) no matter how difficult it is. Anything less than this indicates you are not ready to progress within this ray; it is better to leave it alone.

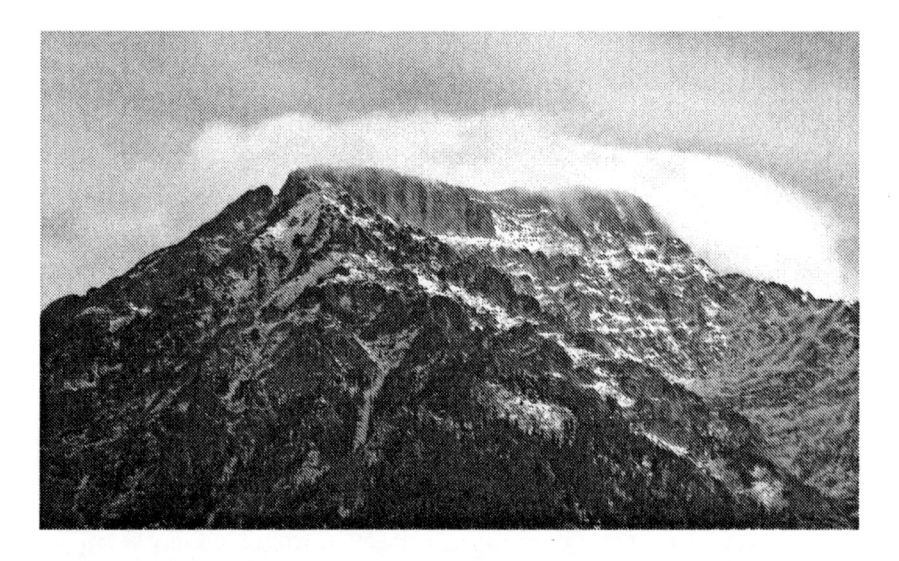

A grounded ability to work through the Silver Ray is an advanced accomplishment. While all of the Ascended Masters work with this ray at various times, Saint Germain and El Morya in particular use it often, as do some of the dragons within the earth.

A few times we have participated in working with the dragons and Masters in grounding Silver Ray activations within a local area. While describing the fullness of this activity is beyond the scope of this book, this is usually done to help prepare the energy for further activity, and to remove certain blockages in the energy field. It is an impersonal activity, although of course, there is always etheric assistance for those who truly want to grow with it. The animals are usually very sensitive to it. This kind of activity will occur much more often as many of the deep masterful beings within the earth, what many would call angels, start to come towards the surface again. While this is occurring, we have witnessed a number of people experiencing difficulties in adjusting to the changes. Some resist change, or try to attack its source (like throwing rocks at the sun), without quite knowing what it is they are resisting. Some become very delusional, feeling the activation and channeling all sorts of non-sense. It is simply a speeding up of people's already existing tendencies. Some become hyperactive and some very internal. If taken within, it is a great opportunity for growth.

While the Silver Ray is not really subject to grosser personality qualifications, as are some of the other rays, if I was to use a single word to describe effects on those who attune to it ignorantly, I would say delusion, or misdirection.

The Silver Ray has an eclectic and electric quality, enhancing communication, telepathy, multiple subtle-body projection, and relocation in space. As a distinct color, it is more evident in the higher realms, particularly the eighth center a few inches above the head.

Proper use of the Silver Ray requires wakefulness and fluidity within all the body-centeRed Rays, which in itself requires you are awake within the central channel. Without this fluidity, the Silver Ray does not have the room it needs to work elastically and as a light. In such a scenario, the Silver Ray becomes more cold, metallic and solid, essentially devoid of any of its true essence—being more a projection of the imagination.

Silver is closely connected to the color blue, and is part of the electrical activity of the Aquamarine and White Rays. The Silver Ray is formed of subtle mind pranas. The scintillating light of silver and gold can easily be created as an activity of the higher-mind, and through skilled connectivity, precipitated into the body as a subtle nourishment. This can be done through drawing it in as a white light sparkling with silver, from just above the head into the center and back of the head. The Silver Ray helps align the pineal gland in the center of the head.

Like Gold, the Silver Ray quickens the metallic ions in the body to a higher vibratory state, so that greater cosmic energies are absorbed into it. This is very helpful in preparing yourself as a greater vehicle of your higher Light. It helps awaken awareness of your light body; you feel it more and see through it more easily; it becomes a tangible quality of your awareness. Activity on the Silver Ray is not something to seek out. It will come to you, through the Masters, as the time is right.

For this working of the Silver Ray, two things must occur. First, through decree and meditation, you sensitize the upper head centers. During this activity, the upward absorption of sexual chemistry is very important, so its nectars can combine with this ray and soften its effects. The sexual chemistry itself is charged with this higher intention. Maintaining semen during sexual intercourse or through celibacy, while important, is not enough. This stream of energy must be directed and contained into opening the higher centers in a way that is only understood through the passion of higher meditation.

For most people, complex healing is needed prior to being able to do this, including intimate, vulnerable relationships. However, at some point, the higher chemistry is recognized. At this point, one no longer grasps onto outer relationship as the source of their power. True relationship is empowered, whole, complete, natural, trusting, and vibrant with a happy sense of being.

In your visualization of silver, do not confuse it with a grey color. The silver is very bright, full of limitless energy, and is of a very refined nature with a whiteness to it. The silver ray, properly understood, has a youthful quality, to it and gives a sense of limitless energy, lightness and a glow to the body.

A very advanced use of the Silver Ray is to make the Ascension suit, whereby the physical body can be brought into the Light and then back into physicality. In this application, the Silver Ray becomes the interface. The adept must already be whole on all the other rays, having overcome all karmic weakness in the body. The silvery-White Ray descending from above infuses itself into the skin, becoming your skin. This skin gives a concentration and definition in the Light through which the aspirant projects themselves as a body of Light. This is a difficult concept to explain. The actual infusion occurs through the central channel. However, the skin is emphasized, because in a way you have become hollow of the need to remain as an individual.

In the Masters' retreats, an adept receives their seamless garment as they are initiated into working with all the rays from the feeling of their One Presence. The seamless garment is a clothing of nectar-light that helps to hold the integrity of the body image in an elevated feeling of light.

To wear the seamless garment an adept has already overcome their physical karmas; however, subtle astral karmas can still be present. As these are overcome and the adept feels home to be the light in which they sit, then the Ascension suit is earned. In this silver skin, one is free to work on the cosmic levels of creation.

Any areas that are not of the karma-free Light in the body simply do not allow the Silver Ray to actualize over that part in its full integrity or stability.

As this silver suit is mastered it becomes all the cells of the body. The silver suit is the causal radiance of the blue flame or cosmic image of your perfected form, sustained by that thought. It is an integration of the Blue Pearl[10] experienced at the pineal gland when the Amrit Nadi[11] is activated. While every cell of your body takes on this radiance, the reason it is called a suit is because it is like wearing a new body, and one that has much greater freedom. The golden

---

[10] The Blue Pearl is nectar, a tangible living light, connected to the fabric of creation. In this, you can experience a more enlightened aspect of yourself, and many other forms within the universe, as easily as you would take a breath. When looking through its ethers, it brings many visions. When fully entered, it is a profound loss of conventional identity, exchanged for the fluidity of consciousness itself experiencing different forms and realities. While incredibly sacred, it is a step towards, not the completion, of the ascended body.

[11] The Amrit Nadi is very blissful and profound awakening of buddhic conscious in the central channel between the head and the heart.

ray of the higher pranas blends through it and shines through it like molten silver and gold swirling through each other, as each other. All the other rays can also take form in this fusion.

I have seen ethereal walls of wrongly qualified silver substance that certain priestly people have intentionally created, from the eighth realm, around particular vortices, temples, and places they use as a source of power. This psychic presence, mostly felt in a mental way to those who are aware of it, is a way of keeping their qualifications upon the local radiations from within the earth predominant. While it can appear cozy to people who want to keep things along certain established lines, it is very stifling to the higher soul activity, and actively shuts things down in terms of true soul growth. A person who is conscious of the Silver Ray can, when appropriate, penetrate into it, see what needs to be seen, and dissolve this ethereal blockage; otherwise, people are left to have their own experiences for a time.

This type of projection is much different from the way a Master will use the Silver Ray for activation, maintaining integrity of a process, and for protection of those within that process. Whenever this activity extends outside of ones immediate body, a Master will work in alignment with the underlying enlightened beings within the earth, and always from a perspective only possible through the Body of the One. A Master will blend with a feminine sensitivity, and is able to work in a fluid manner—not too much, not too little—thus moving as appropriate. Rather than shutting down higher awareness, it is just the opposite. Purposefully disruptive energies are not the enemy, although they can, and often are, returned strongly to themselves.

A word of warning; be very careful of your intentions with this ray. Intentional misuse of it as a detriment to others, or to take what is not yours, has strong kickbacks. Even if you are not checked immediately, it is only a matter of time. While a leeway of ignorance is allowed in the misuse of other rays in how the energy is returned (similar to how leeway is given to children), the misuse of a cosmic ray has much greater consequences. I have seen people exit the planet very quickly and the ramifications can carry forth for many lifetimes.

Decrees

"I AM God in action."

"I AM the clear path to the Beloved Ascended Masters."

Turquoise

Turquoise is a healing, cooling, clear color often associated with the historical Buddha. It is a wonderful activation of the thymus gland above the heart, bringing forth youthfulness and a greater connection to the realms within the earth.

Turquoise is sometimes felt with the dolphin energy in its free-emotional wisdom, as well as with the Devas. It is helpful to meditate with the Turquoise Ray from the eighth chakra above the head along with silver. It brings balance to a predominantly Gold Ray personality. The Turquoise Light harbors Divine wisdom, compassion, helps in clear communication and facilitates a lightness of spirit recognizing the limitless shores of the Ever-Expanding reality of our universe.

Aquamarine

Aquamarine brings forth an electrical vitality of the Blue Ray, giving strength in subtle projection and a rich, watery field of awareness. It naturally co-exists with the Silver and White rays and it enhances the Orange Ray. Meditating with an aquamarine crystal is a good way to get in touch with the Aquamarine Ray.

The Aquamarine Ray functions primarily within the etheric fabric from the eighth center above the head. Its use in the body should primarily be through the central channel, with a natural resonance in the etheric chord emphasizing the second chakra, thymus, and throat.

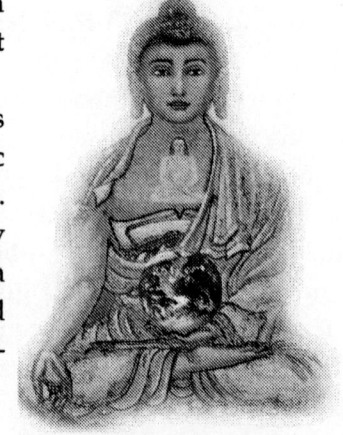

The Aquamarine Ray greatly enhances subtle mental body activity, particularly giving awareness of spatial qualities and dimensions, thereby helping you to connect more tangibly. Meditating with the Aquamarine Ray opens subtle sight and visionary abilities. However, there lies a trap in its premature use. If you are not well rounded in the various rays and connected to your purity, a subtle pride is also generated. Such a person lacks the humility to align fully into the Oneness.

A further misuse of the Aquamarine Ray occurs through a person who is very aware of the telepathic currents among a group of people and will manipulate those currents to their advantage, outwardly supporting the disempowered social behavior that allows their activity to go unnoticed. This can be seen in some souls who develop their inner capacity through meditation, yet hold onto a priestly role of maintaining religious or dharmic activity.

The Aquamarine Ray is very connected to a fluidic nature, like water that has an aura of electrical fire. The nature of this courageous ray breaks down many social barriers that would inhibit a soul from taking its next step. A soul carrying this ray will often "stretch the rules" of what is acceptable to bring forth growth and go into places that others would fear to tread. The person bringing forth new developments in established fields and the political revolutionary who has the interest of the people at heart will often tap into this ray.

Aquamarine brings forth an idealistic nature, a poetic streak and a visionary romance with the subtle. Aquamarine was one of the rays often tapped into by Sri Aurobindo.

Clear Light

Clear Light is as an awareness of radiance. This can occur on many levels, yet the feeling of clarity is common to all, as if everything is more conscious.

It can be as simple as your eyes sparkling. It can be a feeling, which you are suddenly aware of, as if your whole existence is a projection from above or deep within.

The expression, Clear Light, can indicate awareness of a presence that is beyond your ability to perceive, or of a formless nature.

There is an underlying harmony and directness. In its highest reference, the Clear Light refers to awareness within the twelfth realm. It is the very idea of God, the universal sea of possibility and the brightness and perfection always contained within it and available to all souls who align to it. It is not something you evoke; rather, it is something you are when you are in the purity of your truth.

The Clear Light is an activating presence. The support of Clear Light allows you to undertake any service and to undergo any growth that you approach wholeheartedly and without doubt. Every possible phenomena and existence is realized to be a radiant idea in the mind of God. All emotions, forms, and experiences are made up of various primal ideas interacting with each other.

There is nowhere to go, nothing to do. A soul radiating the Clear Light is moving to their home in the Body of the One. There is an incredible underlying sense of simplicity, no matter how complicated life outwardly appears.

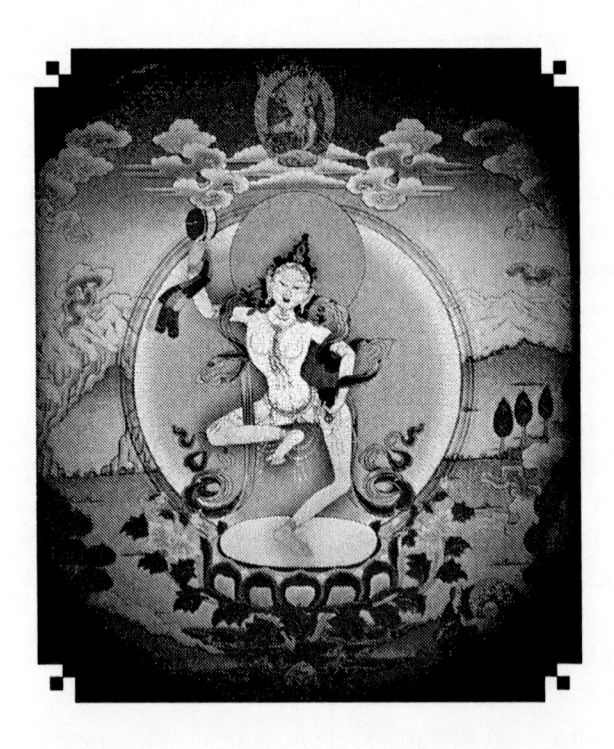

A Quick Summary of the Rays

Ray	Positive Quality	Negative Quality
Blue	Primal Awareness Sharp Mind Loyalty	Righteousness
Violet	Sacred Alchemy Independent Spirit Global Thinking	Arrogance
Gold	Confidence Capable	Ego-centered (willful) Stubborn
Orange	Transformative	Impulsive Self Destructive tendencies Over Indulgence
	Consistent Strength Handles Pressure well	Power Crazy Insensitive
Pink	Compassion, Forgiveness Softness	Naïve Manipulation Uses Other People for Strength
White	Nectar	Prideful
Silver	Bridging	Misdirecting
Green	Connectivity Harmonious Eloquent	Covert (deceptive) Hidden Agenda

DAILY PRACTICE AND ESTABLISHING A RETREAT

Importance of Establishing a Foundational Practice Prior to Beginning Eternal Yoga

Prior to beginning the practices within this book, a routine of daily spiritual practices needs to be well-established. More than writing in a journal or moments of self-reflection, this routine should include dynamic transformative activities, by which you can move energy and continually return to a place of vital balance and clarity. This daily routine should include deep meditative movements through both quiet absorption and active focus, such as within the kriyas.

The book, Cultivating a Body of Nectar: Kriya Yoga and Tantric Foundations (see appendix) is filled with practices and advice for establishing a daily practice. Those who are sincere may consider coming to our retreat center (see appendix) to receive further instruction, and perhaps to live in the student's practice house for a period to better establish themselves in the art of developing an effective daily practice. This creates the foundation by which further advancement can occur. We have seen again and again, that without this foundation and the habit of going within yogically to move through potentially growthful moments, even with the best of initial intentions, people get stuck. During challenging situations, what should be taken within, becomes externalized into all the reasons why not to change, or something someone else is doing to us.

While these are very potent practices for those who are ready, there is no quick fix. The fastest route is a consistent application spiced by the passion to penetrate into our divine depth, the courage to apply this to our own growth, and the surrender to release false ambitions and stuckness. When you truly engage in a yogic practice, you experience not only elevating moments, but also purification. It takes substance to apply ourselves through this purification.

As you are ready to begin the practices of Eternal Yoga, understand that this is a type of tantric initiation. Let go of any misconceptions around the concept of what tantra is, such as sex, sensations, blending, etc. Tantra is developing the continuum of our awareness, including all facets of life, from within the core of our body. If this core is not awakened to a level of buddhic awareness, then it is not tantra. Eternal Yoga is an opportunity to enter into this depth, and in this context it is an initiatory beginning in which the tantras can commence.

One of the reasons Eternal Yoga is an entry into the tantras is that a connection with the body is always maintained within the practice of buddhic activation. While this is a preliminary into later tantric practices, which emphasizes a centering within the inner core of the body, it will, in a tantric fashion, greatly stimulate subtle attitudes and karmas into physical manifestation. Without a yogic foundation, it is unlikely that you will be able to apply yourself in an effective manner through this, and will simply get lost in the rapidly changing landscape. Instead of growth, you will most likely fall back into old ways of interaction and miss the opportunity of releasing yourself from the wheel. These practices, when purely applied, will change how you see everything. This way of seeing is a tantric activity.

While a yogic foundation greatly benefits from the guidance of a competent teacher(s), the tantric path is a disaster without it. While we all have many teachers in this grand union of life, a tantric teacher is a rare occurrence. This is not only a person with whom you have (or will develop) an eternal connection with and who is activated on a buddhic level, but without the slightest hesitation, he or she understands the difference between liberation in the realms of the soul and from a level of spirit. Yet, even this is not enough. As a path of self-initiation, without your own intensity, sincerity, and purity of application then there is no one to blame for becoming lost, but yourself.

One of the benefits of an effective daily practice is that it clears out much of the personality traits that would block the intimate and real connection with a teacher, allowing a clear path of transmission and relationship. Until you gain familiarity with your own non-verbal depth, it is difficult to experience it with another. While I hope that this book inspires you, I do want to discourage you from jumping into its practices until you have done some of the preliminary preparation. Even if you have had a spiritual orientation for several decades, please, first establish an effective and consistent daily practice.

Establishing a Daily Practice of Eternal Yoga

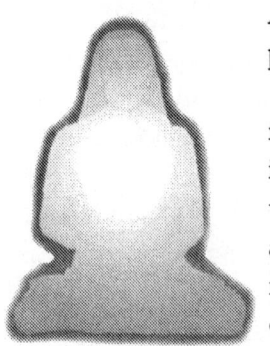

After your initial sincere introduction to these practices,[1] there comes a steady application.

The details of this will look a little different for each person, and the circumstances in which the application is occurring. Keeping up a foundational daily practice, as discussed above, is paramount. Some days will primarily involve Eternal Yoga practices, and some days will involve only a brief touching in above the head with the remaining consisting of your regular foundational practices, such as kriya, yoga, etc.

At the beginning of every practice session, even if you are just doing a yoga set, start by tuning in, go above the head for a moment, and see if there is anything requiring your attention. When you finish a session, if there is any understanding you wish to carry forth from one session to the next, then go a few feet above the head, crystallize the understanding with the intention that you will notice it when you tune in at the beginning of your next session. It is like sticky notes you place on your desk as reminders for when you return. This is much more effective than writing down a written note, for all the subtleties will again present themselves to you. Also be sure to give a heart-felt thanks and blessings for the benefit of another and/or for the benefit of all beings.

---

[1] I recommend attending an intensive with us to get a fuller understanding of the practices, even if you have already started the Eternal Yoga practices from this book. See Appendix for further information.

Developing a continuum from each practice session to the next, through methods such as the proceeding paragraph, cannot be overemphasized. It can easily make ten to a hundred times difference over the years in the speed at which you advance. Part of developing this continuum includes the radiant giving of blessings, such as the dedication. By bringing the movement of your practice into a larger energy field beyond your immediate personality, i.e., for the benefit of many beings, you are giving it a greater continuum. This sharing of the heart tends to carry forth throughout the day, transforming you and others around you through the presence of love.

The little moments during the day contribute greatly to keeping your practice alive, such as a remembrance, being consciously conscious while you are doing something, and dwelling in your radiant depth and breath. Even a minute, or a few seconds here and there, is extremely beneficial. Even if we meditate one, two, five, eight hours a day, there are still many hours of the day that we are not engaged in meditation. If during these hours we always forget and allow our old habits to enforce their position, then we are always fighting an uphill battle. The little moments are what make the difference, and in time, this will allow a new perspective to gain a solid foothold. This new perspective becomes the dominant view, the natural state. Having a radiant core of energy in your body activated to a buddhic depth is like having a gentle hand on your shoulder. You do not have to try to remember, it is always there. In this way you are not just having a passing spiritual experience, rather you are that which never sleeps, enjoying the ever-changing experience.

There will be periods of a few months where you are intensely involved in activity above your head and it dominates both your sitting practice and many moments during the day. All of that activity above the head can create a spacey quality. It is sometimes beneficial for a while, but not for too long of a duration. Thus, you will have periods of a few months when it is important to shift the emphasis clearly within the body. This can involve focusing on a whole body feeling, or perhaps within a particular chakra or quality, such as nectar, a ray, or a character trait.

At times, the intense movement of energy above the head can create headaches or soreness of the scalp. In the beginning weeks of your practice, this is similar to getting sore muscles—it will disappear as you become accustomed to a greater flow of energy through the top of the head. When you finish your practice, be sure to bring the energy down into the body, particularly the navel area, and feel a wholesome balance. Some exercise and stretching helps.

There are times when you might get a headache because something requires your attention above the head, or you might become internal, similar to a tired feeling. The headache or tired feeling will often quickly disappear when you stop, perhaps lie down, and totally go into it, seeing what you need to see. In this type of scenario, you have to look in the right place; it is similar to being a detective. If going above your head, or in your body does not give you the vision, then try going down into the earth.

Another source of headaches and aches in the body resulting from practice above the head occurs when you are bringing in a cosmic ray or understanding and you are not grounding it correctly. You may be throwing it around in the outer channels, instead of containing and centering it deep within the central core of the body and letting it intelligently and softly radiate out from there. Alternatively, you may be receiving something but not applying it. For example, an action may be required, such as speaking out, moving energy in the body, making a change in your life, or making a determined effort to penetrate further into a core understanding. In this scenario, until you engage yourself in the activity, the energy is not flowing. While subtle, the strength of energy-consciousness brought in from above the head can be intense in its ability to make itself felt, not only in you, but in the larger area as well. This cosmic fire is beyond the immediate personality, and as such, requires a consciousness, if you wish to partake of it.

If your energy is too hot in a mental way, this can result in headaches, discomfort, and stagnation. This is usually reflective of a lack of nectar in the head centers often combined with too much intellectual activity. While a rigorous physical workout can help, it will not teach you to solve the problem at its source. The solution is to soften the energy and get out of the thinking mind in this manner. First, do some stretches and breath into the lower part of the body. Then focus in one of the head centers, such as the third eye, and breathe in soft, white light to that center. Give the light a sensual, liquid quality. Also, feel liquid light moving up through your body. While unwaveringly maintaining a focus—relax, and allow the energy to open, becoming more spacious and giving somewhere for energy to move into. Dissolve any thoughts into the liquid, nonverbal, tangible sense of the light. This understanding is part of your foundational practice.

You can greatly facilitate nectar within the body by not wasting sexual energy. For both men and women this involves opening a circulation of energy into all the spaces of the body. For men, this gives an ability to maintain their seed during sex while simultaneously sharing the energy and opening their hearts in love. For women, this results in containment within their blending, experiencing love as and far beyond the personality. Of course, there is a lot of self-discovery to occur in obtaining this mastery, including refinement, emotional maturity, and spiritual discovery. We need to first find intimacy and mastery within ourselves; this is often best supported through celibacy. There are many aspects of lifestyle, including diet, work, and environment that all play their part in building a deep, supportive energy within our body.

The ins and outs of life itself—relationship, work, kids—are all part of our spiritual discovery, joy, and application. While you will most likely have to make some clear boundaries to assist your discipline, it is important that your practice does not become a means of escape. The spiritual path is truly an intense application and experience that reflects into and through all aspects of your life. Alternatively, all aspects of your life reflect into your spiritual practice.

As you advance, it is easy to be aware of many things at once without losing a feeling of simplicity. This is a quality of the Body of the One. There is not a searching, or mental effort involved at all. For example, you can be outside doing yard work and at the same time aware of certain radiations, communications, and events occurring in the subtle realms. You might stop for a few moments to be present within those realms, and then continue with the enjoyment of working outside.

Another example of this effortless simultaneous awareness is while speaking, perhaps seemingly mundane words, you are aware of addressing and interacting with not only those in front of you, but other beings not present, and even other moments in the future of those whom you are talking with. You are aware of the effects of your actions and presence on many levels. When this occurs in a natural simplicity, it allows us to be aware of, and present to the moment at hand in a manner not otherwise possible.

Retreats

While a daily practice integrated into a wholesome lifestyle is necessary, periods of intensive spiritual application are required for reaching that which is otherwise always just around the corner.

There are many approaches to retreat, reflective of our current ability and situation. Some people look upon retreat as a type of vacation where they get time-out to read a novel, sleep in, meditate, go for walks, and de-stress. By the time the retreat is over, they are ready to jump back into the ambition of the work-world, refreshed and keen for more. For our purposes, this is not what we mean by retreat, although some of these benefits are an added bonus.

Spiritual retreat is a focused intensive application during which we absorb ourselves into a wakeful state that is beyond the confines of our previous conditioning. While purifying ourselves of mundane involvements and becoming captivated in the joy of our penetration, we enter into a beautiful, timeless, simplicity of the heart. We let go of our traditional ways of identification and getting strength to discover ourselves in a new light. Retreat, properly done, is a life-transforming experience. You will never be the same again.

A retreat helps to keep your practice from becoming mundane. For those who apply themselves under our direction, we require at least one retreat a year of a minimum of two weeks. This is a minimum; a more optimal time would be four to six weeks. In addition, a number of shorter, intensive applications are of benefit. Occasionally, the necessity and desire for longer retreats of three months to several years becomes self-evident.

While sometimes an experienced practitioner will spontaneously enter into a retreat; for example, starting tomorrow morning, generally you prepare for a retreat. Often this begins a month before, with longer sittings, prayers and intentions of setting the energy, etc. While, from one perspective, a retreat is always going into the deep-end, in that sense you can never be "prepared" for it. From another perspective, you do prepare yourself by fortifying your intention, gradually increasing your meditative ability, purifying your diet, and looking forward to it. We accumulate a voltage that we can use within the retreat itself. During the retreat, this accumulated voltage will help us to rise up earlier, to sit more alertly, and to keep going through difficulties. When we might otherwise fall back into an old pattern, something inside of us reminds us why we are on retreat, and we snap back into our forward movement. Because we have set the energy from the start, we can do this with one movement, rather than a lot of jerky stops and starts.

It is important that we create a retreat situation that is practical for our ability, thus not originating from fantasyland. This is where an experienced guide can help you. If you can only sit for thirty minutes before your knees give out, then do not expect suddenly be able to sit for four hours at a stretch. You have to work up to these things. However, it is within reason to extend this time to an hour. Do not instantly think you will only need to sleep two hours per day—there is a lot of integration that occurs. For some it may be too much not to have some stimulation from reading, so in that case allow one or two appropriate books that are directly beneficial to your retreat. At the same time, set limits. Forget TV, radio, the newspaper, your cup of coffee, phone calls, and trips into town. Keep food simple, of sufficient nourishment, and easy. Do include walks in nature, naps, etc. Decide ahead of time who you will interact with; for example, your teacher, a person bringing you food, perhaps a phone call once per week to your kids. In terms of your practice, there are set practices and there has to be room for the unfolding of the retreat itself to show you what is needed.

Setting up an altar is the first activity of your retreat. Then sit down, intensely focus upon your intention, speak it aloud, and create the boundaries of your retreat.

Following is an example of a typical retreat day:

- *Meditation, typically starting several hours before sunrise*
- *A short break, perhaps some tea and fruit*
- *Morning yoga set*
- *Meditation*
- *Lunch*
- *Walk in nature*
- *Afternoon meditation*
- *Dinner*
- *Evening practice, such as a kriya followed by meditation*
- *Sleep*
- *Possibly a session during the late night*

Be sure to include short naps when needed. Keep the energy fresh. Do not be hesitant to stretch in the middle of a meditation session. This is a very general guideline. For example, an advanced practitioner may meditate straight through from the early morning hours until near lunchtime. Another may have shorter meditation sessions and much of the retreat is the letting go of need for external stimulation and learning how to be with one's self.

While most retreats are a solo experience, small group retreats can, if well structured, give the benefit of a group structure to aid in application, energy, and discipline. This works particularly well if everyone is sincere and supportive of each other. This support should not become a social structure of chitchat and drawing emotionally on one another. Of course, there are occasional exceptions in times of circumstance, but in general, a retreat is not a commune. Silence should be the norm, and each person established in his or her own energy.

You are creating a Divine field of energy, sourced beyond the personality, and potentized through each involved. This can be challenging, because as this divine stimulation enters into the personality, issues needing to become cleared can find a way to polarize between group participants. Skillfully and quickly recognizing the underlying issues can bring to attention our blind spots and thereby stimulate growth. I emphasize quickly, because if a retreat situation becomes instead one long therapy session, then while the emotional self may feel some movement, the subtle fabric of the retreat is broken, and the potential of the retreat to discover and cultivate oneself beyond this framework of personality has been lost. Within these scenarios, each member needs to find a way to apply themselves in accordance with the sincerity of their retreat intentions. Sometimes learning how to create this dynamic becomes the principle teaching of the retreat for those involved.

Men and women together in retreat can work well and create a more balanced energy field, provided there is latitude for differences in application. Men and woman will work differently in how they apply themselves in practice. Particularly women need and will demand more breathing space in the scope of their application. This is because of the greater scope required for woman to work with their inherently stronger alchemy of emotions including the influence of cycles and the perfections within each phase of a cycle. If a woman can use this energy as a support, then it is a great aid. It is not a one rule fits all. Some men are blind to this, and the enthusiasm of their retreat practice, if projected onto a woman as the man's need for a rigid support structure, can quickly make things unworkable. In regards to a retreat with a man and woman, there should be celibacy, unless the retreat is specifically using the energy of lovemaking as part of the spiritual practice, and it is easy for the man to contain his seed.

Generally, four hours is the absolute maximum time between practice sessions, with an exception at night for those who truly need the extra sleep. Be sure to rise early, before sunrise. Much of a retreat involves increasing familiarity with deep non-verbal and connected states. For this, you must have a proper balance of mind, that is, there is just the right level of firmness. If your mind constantly needs outer activity and cannot rest in stillness, then you need a combination of kriyas to channel this energy into stillness, along with longer sittings in which we find ourselves beyond the outer levels of definition. While in our daily practice we may have relied more on active kriyas (such as pranayama) and dynamic movement for this function, in retreat we need to learn how to do this innately, and thus we rely more on longer sittings that are more passive in nature than kriyas. In longer sittings, we can cultivate an inner support, such as through the breathless nectars.

If you become vacant, unconscious, tranquil, and unresponsive within your meditation and during the day in general, then you have lost this balance. While occasionally we have to go into this imbalance in order to release the need for the ego to always be in control, do not let this become a habit - include active practices, such as dynamic yoga sets, pranayama, and kriya. Provide enough time for integration, such as naps and walks. Nature herself helps to bring us into balance and is a tremendous source of teaching, healing, and inspiration. You may develop a friendship with a favorite tree or an opening by a stream.

A retreat is a special opportunity to enter into the experience of emptiness. For many, this can initially be an uncomfortable experience, and thus there is avoidance in getting too deep into this during our previous daily practice. It just does not appear to fit with the demands of daily life or our ambitions and mode of self-definition. This is often an uncomfortable experience, like the fear of death. In releasing the force of our grasping at our individuality, we experience a kind of death. In that expansion, we can feel a bit lost. Through the special circumstances of a retreat, we can more easily let go of these outer considerations, such as the need to hold everything together through the force of our personality. Becoming more familiar with this depth beyond ownership of our personality, we let go of our unfounded fears, and start to enjoy it. We learn that emptiness is not a vacuum, or lack, rather a very direct experience of all that is. There is a richness and opening of the heart. We become more fearless and relaxed in just being who we are. We begin to know ourselves within the true nature of reality.

In regards to the Eternal Yoga practice, a retreat is the perfect opportunity to go for it. You can meditate above your head for hours at a time. You can make a determined effort, a decree, to see what you need to see, and with the continual penetration of your decree, actually see what you need to see. A day of this can equal a year or more of mundane practice. Through the hours of application, you can gain greater inner definition. It is extremely important that in this kind of intense application within the buddhic realms, that you find a thread within everything you see and experience that returns you to yourself for further growth. What is your part in what you see? Why are you seeing this? How did you create this?

In this way, you not only find your blind spots, but also empower yourself into another level of responsibility and identification. You are not just trying to polish another facet of your existence; rather, you are overcoming the root ignorance that keeps you bound. You are shifting into a completely new way of seeing things. This is more than a different angle of perception, rather, a release from the solidity of illusion itself. This transparency brings forth awareness of the Body of the One. The Body of the One is not just a collective mish-mash of thoughts and emotions, for this awareness by itself would simply result in our insanity. The Body of the One is a conscious awareness within the oneness of those awakened as source itself. What you are finding is the operation of your Ever-Expanding Perfection, and in that, the same for all of creation.

There is perhaps no better way to deepen dream yoga, than in a retreat situation. Unless you are specifically gearing the retreat for dream recall through its structure, your first days may be devoid of dreams. That is, you may be going out beyond where you can recall. However, this will likely shift. The clarity generated through a retreat application cannot help but to enter into your dream life as well. This is not only about vivid dreaming, but also, perhaps your first experiences of staying awake, without dreaming, while the body sleeps.

After you have mastered the understandings of Eternal Yoga, and receive the blessings of the Masters, you are able to enter into tantric retreats. This includes periods of specialized work within the earth, dark retreats, consort retreat practice, and advanced nectar cultivation resulting in siddhas. A dark retreat is a specialized advanced retreat, traditionally done for six to seven weeks by those who are able. Otherwise, a week is good. This type of retreat occurs in a pitch-black environment, with no external contact other than with your teacher. A further enhancement is to do the retreat in a specially prepared room within the earth. This type of retreat develops internal vision, cuts through illusory identification, and brings regeneration if this is one of the aims of the retreat. For success, you must already have developed enough internal definition to provide a firmness of mind independent of the body, while at the same time also having a non-verbal energetic awareness within the body that you can easily rest in for long periods.

In a retreat, you can build the prana within various centers of your body to support greater consciousness. This is a cultivation of the nectars. These nectars support greater awareness above the head, and the simultaneous integration of that buddhic light within the body. Building these nectars is one of the reasons to let go of too much mental activity. Leave the laptop at home. Too much analytical activity is a fire that can burn up these nectars before they have the chance to build sufficiently.

A retreat is not just an initiation into a new way of being; it is practice within that new way of being. Thus, retreats are very practical. For someone who has never been able to release the chitchat of their mind, a successful retreat of a month may involve first gaining this ability, then remaining in it for the remainder of the retreat. This will give that person not only an experience, but also the expertise to come back into this ease repeatedly long after the retreat has finished. You have gained a stepping-stone for further growth. As the retreat draws to a close, you may gain glimpses of what lies ahead of you, now achievable through this new ability.

Retreats are not always just about ourselves. Sometimes, you initiate a retreat primarily for the purpose of service, such as developing and holding a particular blessing presence within the earth, praying for the betterment of a world situation, etc. For those who are able, this is a wonderful type of retreat to enter into. In participating in the bigger picture, whatever of ourselves that gets in the way, we will be motivated to purify that. In this type of retreat, because we are participating in the bigger picture, we will naturally come into further contact with the Masters and angels who also participate in the bigger picture as their life blood.

Especially in longer retreats, there develops an awareness of the Perfection and the Masters meditating you. A retreat is a great opportunity to develop a connection with one or more of the Ascended Masters. This connection becomes the heart of your very existence, there is a tremendous level of trust and oneness. The more you enter within the stillness of your own self, the more this relationship with the Masters develops, which further fuels the desire to enter deeper into yourself.

In regards to a retreat of several months to several years, one of the Masters usually initiates this. The Masters themselves are bringing you in, when you are ready. Effortless long periods of sitting, are again, usually the result of one of the Masters bringing you further into this level of absorption. You are entering far beyond the limits of what the immediate personality can decree or do. You can pray for this and do your part in becoming ready.

You cannot achieve a successful retreat through sheer force of egoic determination. It requires a level of support. This support comes from friends who look after things while you are gone and make sure you have food. This support comes from the earth and from local spirits. It comes from the giving you share through blessings while on retreat. It comes from the Masters, and it comes from your own Higher-Self activated by the sincerity of your intention and the call of your passion.

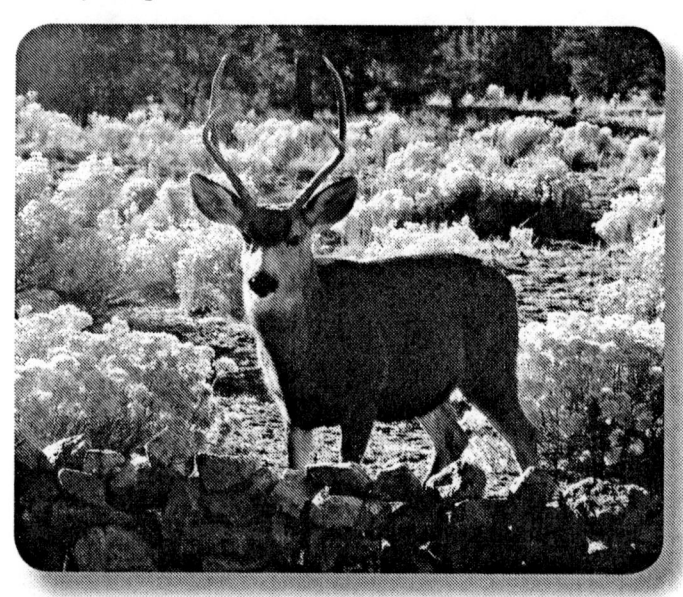

Cultivating a Body of Nectar: *Kriya Yoga and Tantric Foundations*

by Virochana Khalsa
ISBN 1-929952-04-X
288 pages $21.95

Skillfully presented in this book are numerous methods to develop our blissful body of nectar.

After introducing an overview of the process, the author proceeds into specifics, This well illustrated book includes an extensive section on meditative techniques known as kriyas.

Virochana also explains, in his typical radiant wisdom, detailed understandings of chakras, channels, energy and essences through which we can create an inner temple.

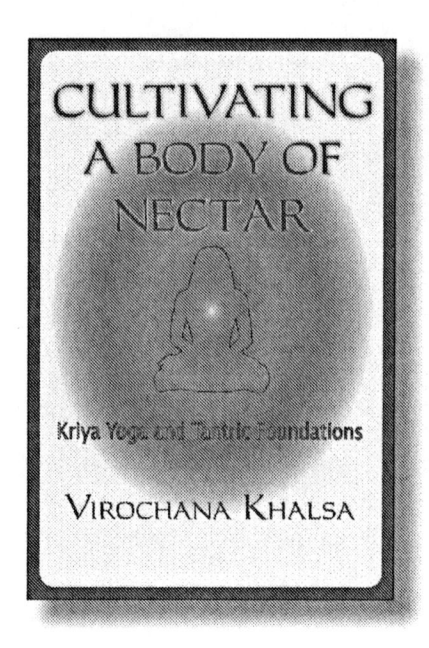

"Through our blissful affair with cultivating nectar, we know our spirit in form...
Creating a body of nectar is an artful science that any of us can master through a steady, sincere and courageous application."

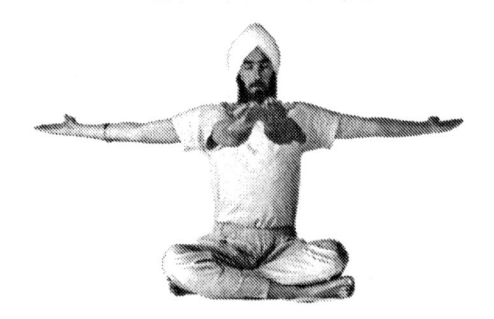

Tantra Unveiled, through the feminine

by Whitecloud Khalsa
ISBN 1-929952-03-1
144 pages $14.95

Tantra is a sacred doorway to the secret teachings, opened by mystics who embrace Divine Union.

The revelations and wisdom imparted in this book are from an experienced yogini. Whitecloud received the essence of Tantra from her first Master in India as a young woman, and has further developed this path with the assistance of numerous ascended Masters and her Twin-Ray.

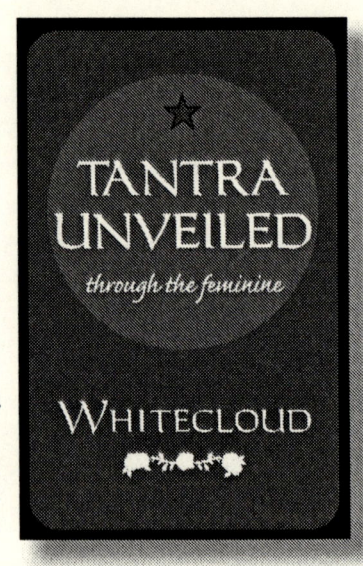

This book is invaluable for anyone wanting to know the totality of what Tantra is as a spiritual path.

> From the day I arrived my master drew me into his intimate radiance. He could make my fever rise and lower by the intensity of his attention towards me, all of which was on a non-verbal level. This force of love blissfully immobilized me. There were no questions within me; instinctively I knew my entire karmic residue was being purified in the fire of kundalini, all the dross being burned in the fever and I only knew love.

The Way of the Goddess, A Journey of Self Awakening

By Shantara Ma Khalsa
(aka Whitecloud)
ISBN 0-9598048-3-8
224 pages $11.95

An exciting, easy to read and transformational biography of her trials, difficulties and victories in her spiritual path and the quest to meet her beloved. Selected by the New Zealand International Woman's Book Festival.

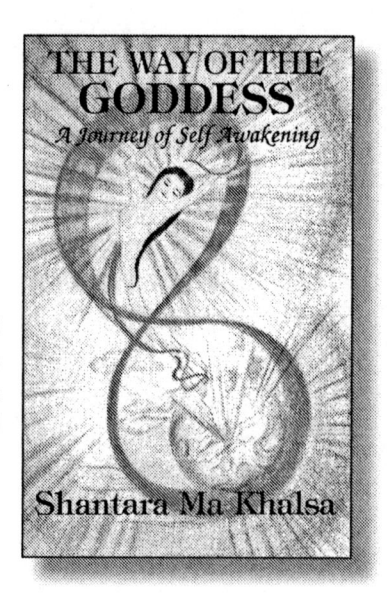

"The teaching of the Eternal Beloved Twin Ray relationship is one of the most important understandings for all souls on the earth today. The coming together of the Twin Ray Flame is achieved after individual enlightenment is attained. The amount of Light and cosmic power focused through this embodied relationship is greater than any individual can ever project."

Resurrection of Earth and Human

By Whitecloud
ISBN 1-929952-07-4
68 pages $12.95

Our earth is an evolving living form. She is encoded with the capacity to cleanse away all that causes her dis-ease. We the Human who have the ears to hear and courage to change must listen to her voice or we will not survive the coming changes. This booklet written at the request of the Ascended Masters Lord Meru and Mu, is for the Hu-man voices for change, voices for peace.

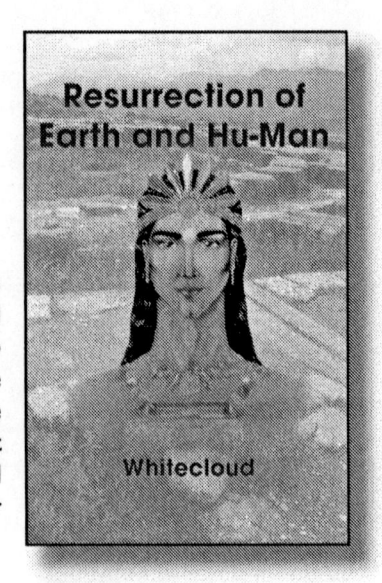

Coming Soon
Look on the web site www.sacredmountainretreat.org
for new books and videos.

Tantra as a Complete Path
by Virochana Khalsa

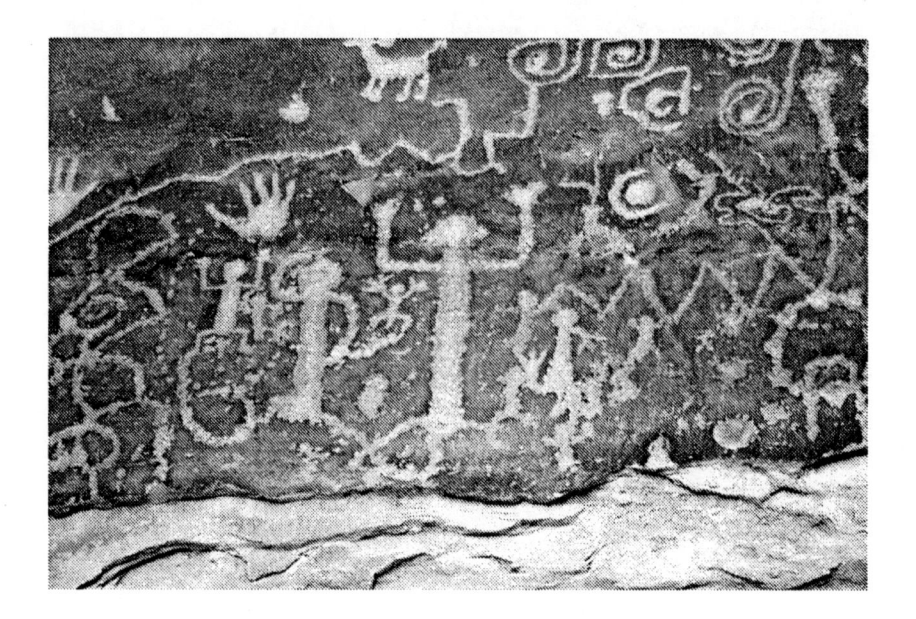

"Non-dual nature is getting there by being there. For example, say you want clarification or guidance on some concern and go within for this purpose. If your mind is in a question mode, a "what if" mode, then you are open to all sorts of frequencies. Your mind could manufacture what you want to hear, or some influence in left field could say what it wants.

The non-dual approach is to first establish yourself in clarity, then expand your knowingness to understand the answer. Thus you first decree, "I AM Clarity." "I AM the clarity of whatever I want to know." However long it takes to establish this feeling, this alignment within yourself, is the inner work necessary to receive the knowingness of your answer.

In meditation practice, non-dual nature does not seek with the mind. In a chant, you are not trying to put together the meaning of the mantra, rather, you are deepening your vibratory presence with the mantra in a nonverbal centering. Yoga practice is thus a deepening of being there.

In non-dual nature you do not look to the techniques as your liberation, rather you simply use them to deepen your already known Presence. This simple understanding has very profound ramifications. Surprising as it may seem, many on the yogic path seem to miss it."

from Tantra of the Beloved - Virochana

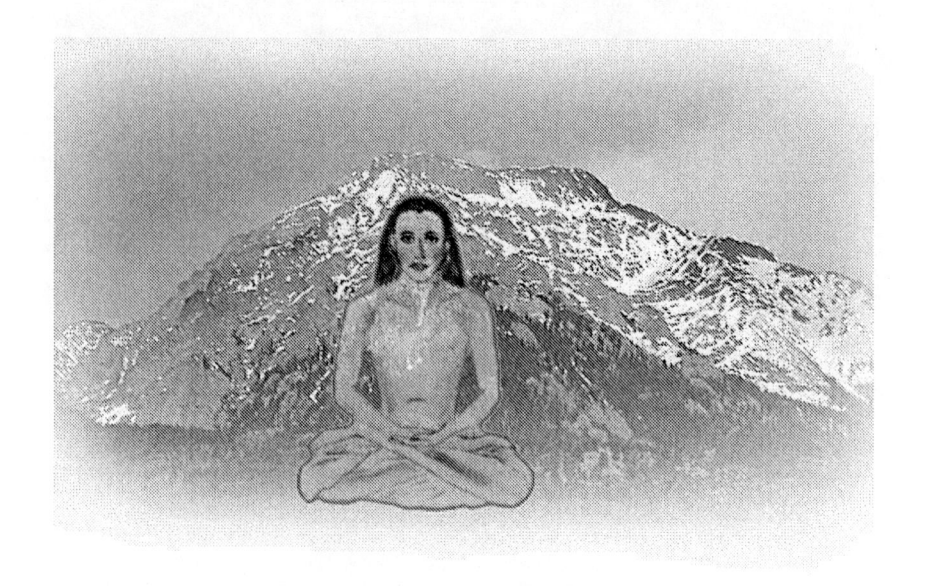